Pediatric Otology

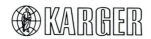

Volume Editors
C. Cremers, Nijmegen
G. Hoogland, Plasmolen-Mook

36 figures, 1 color plate and 40 tables, 1988

KARGER

Basel · München · Paris · London · New York · New Delhi · Singapore · Tokyo · Sydney

Advances in Oto-Rhino-Laryngology

Library of Congress Cataloging-in-Publication Data
International Symposium on Pediatric Otology (1987: Nijmegen, The Netherlands)
Pediatric otology/International Symposium on Pediatric Otology,
Nijmegen, April 23–25, 1987; volume editors, C. Cremers, G. Hoogland.
(Advances in oto-rhino-laryngology; vol. 40)
Includes bibliographies and index.
1. Pediatric otology-Congresses.
I. Cremers, C. W. R.J. (Cornelius Wilhelmus Radboud Jozef), 1945– .
II. Hoogland, G. A.   III. Title.   IV. Series.
[DNLM: 1. Ear Diseases – in infancy & childhood-congresses.
W1 AD701 v. 40/WV 200 I617p 1987]
RF16.A38 vol. 40 [RF 122.5.C4] 618.92′0977-dc19
DNLM/DLC
ISBN 3–8055–4726–9

Bibliographic Indices
This publication is listed in bibliographic services, including Current Contents® and
Index Medicus.

Drug Dosage
The authors and the publisher have exerted every effort to ensure that drug selection and dosage set forth in this text are in accord with current recommendations and practice at the time
of publication. However, in view of ongoing research, changes in government regulations, and
the constant flow of information relating to drug therapy and drug reactions, the reader is
urged to check the package insert for each drug for any change in indications and dosage and
for added warnings and precautions. This is particularly important when the recommended
agent is a new and/or infrequently employed drug.

Pediatric Otology

Advances in Oto-Rhino-Laryngology

Vol. 40

Series Editor
C.R. Pfaltz, Basel

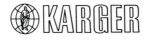

Basel · München · Paris · London · New York · New Delhi · Singapore · Tokyo · Sydney

Contents

Cholesteatoma

Introduction

From the 23rd to the 25th of April, 1987, an International Symposium on Pediatric Otology was held in Nijmegen, The Netherlands. This meeting was part of the continuing activities of the European Working Group in Pediatric Otorhinolaryngology and was hosted by the Department of Otorhinolaryngology, Nijmegen University. Joint sessions were held with The Netherlands Society for Otorhinolaryngology and Cervicofacial Surgery. Congenital aural atresia, serous otitis media and cholesteatoma in children were the main topics covered.

This volume of *Advances in Oto-Rhino-Laryngology* comprises most of the invited papers on these main topics. They provide not only new information but also present the state of the art of these diseases in children.

In our opinion, also other otological diseases in children have to be the subject of our constant attention and scientific work. This book condenses one of the efforts to stimulate progress in our knowledge in the field of pediatric otology.

The editors are much indebted to the speakers for their contributions and especially for the efforts to make their work available for publication in this volume of *Advances in Oto-Rhino-Laryngology*. The editors are most grateful for the help and advice from Mrs. Greder of the Karger Publishing Co. The most hectic moments of the organization of this symposium were mastered by Mrs. Yolanda Hennink and Mrs. Gerry Westerlaken. Finally it should be mentioned that the organization of this symposium was supported by many sponsors. Financial support of the Duphar Company was of great help for the editors in publishing this volume.

Cor Cremers
Gerrit Hoogland

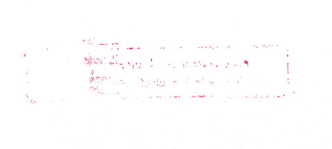

Adv. Oto-Rhino-Laryng., vol. 40, pp. 1–8 (Karger, Basel 1988)

Surgery for Congenital Aural Atresia
The Tübingen Study

Klaus Jahnke, Martin Schrader

Department of Otorhinolaryngology, University of Tübingen, Tübingen, FRG

Classification

Different causes of malformation, as in (a) exogenic malformations, e.g. thalidomide induced; (b) malformations of multifactorial origin, i.e. a combination of genetic and exogenic factors, or (c) monogenic malformations (e.g. Apert-syndrome), imply that any classification of a congenital anomaly must be more or less artificial. There is not always a definite relationship between the severity of malformations of the auricle, the external auditory canal and middle ear. Nevertheless, a classification is justified for preoperative purposes, as case selection and surgical planning, as well as for postoperative evaluation of different techniques, performed in different departments. With these qualifications in mind, we propose to use the classification of Altmann [1955] as a basis. This should be supplemented and subclassified according to preoperative (e.g. missing stapes) and intraoperative findings (e.g. fixed stapes). This means subclassification should preferably depend on the pathology limiting the surgical success, i.e. the pathology of the labyrinthine window region. This contrasts in part with the subclassification of Cremers et al. [1984]. The different degree of outer auditory canal atresia does not influence our indication for surgery.

Type I cases are mostly combined with slight anomalies of the auricle. They are characterized by (a) a small, stenotic external auditory canal, (b) a small tympanic membrane with a short or missing handle of malleus, while in some cases the external auditory canal ends bluntly at the atretic plate level, and (c) an aerated middle ear with ossicles, often a fixed malleus-incus mass connected with a mobile stapes.

In some cases, a type I malformation of the external auditory canal is combined with a fixed or absent stapes, and severe deformities of the labyrinthine windows – especially in patients with mandibulofacial dysostosis. These cases which are unfavorable in respect to the footplate are subclassified as I_s (= severe stapes) cases.

In type II cases microtia or aplasia of the auricle are frequent. They are defined by (a) an atretic external auditory canal – most often over the entire length of the canal; (b) an atretic plate, and (c) an aerated middle ear of normal or smaller size, mostly with a fixed malleus-incus mass but usually a mobile stapes. This is the most common type of major ear malformation. A pathological condition in the footplate region, e.g. facial nerve on oval window, fixed stapes, would result in subclassification II_s.

The type III malformations of Altmann are distinguished from type II in that the tympanic cavity is severely hypoplastic or missing. The ossicles are rudimentary or absent. Frequently, the oval and/or round window cannot be detected and/or the course of the facial nerve is abnormal, e.g. across the oval window niche or the promontory.

Similar thoughts were published by de la Cruz et al. [1985]. Their terms minor and major are confusing, because they are used to differentiate the combined malformations of the external and middle ear on the one hand, and solely of the middle ear on the other. Additionally, malformations of the inner ear should not be included.

Timing of Diagnostic Procedures

Parents of an infant born with unilateral or bilateral major ear malformation usually consult us within the first few days or months of the infant's life. The timing of various diagnostic procedures for children with bilateral major ear malformations is particularly important. As is well known, objective audiometric examinations, such as brain stem audiometry, can be performed in the first months of life. Management with a hearing aid, therefore, is possible at this time. In the first years of life, Stenvers' radiographs of the petrous bone, for example, are indicated only in cases of unclear inner ear function.

When management with a hearing aid is satisfactory, one should wait until the child is older (4–6 years of age) before performing further radiological investigations. In recent years, high-resolution computerized to-mography of the petrous bone, has become the method of choice.

The CT scan should be made directly before surgery, particularly since further advances in noninvasive imaging methods with lower radiation loads are to be expected, for example computer-assisted three-dimensional reconstructions. Conventional tomography should be avoided. A new brain stem audiometry study can be done at the same time. The CT scan provides information not only to the degree of pneumatization, but also on the presence of a malleus-incus conglomerate, the development of the stapes and the inner ear windows, as well as the course of the facial nerve [Jahrsdoerfer et al., 1985].

Timing of Surgery

Surgery for bilateral atresia of the external auditory canal should be performed at 5 or 6 years of age. Surgical treatment of younger patients is justified only if infection is present, for example in cholesteatomas, or when management with a hearing aid has been unsuccessful. Surgery itself and the immediate postoperative phase present no special problems in younger children.

However, difficulties can arise with respect to postoperative care of the newly-created auditory canal and from the middle ear infections that are more frequently associated with Eustachian tube problems at this age.

With grade 1 microtia, that is, with a lesser degree of deformity, uni-lateral creation of an auditory canal and surgery to improve hearing are done at preschool age. At this time the auricle is not operated on.

In patients with grade 2 microtia, intervention for hearing improve-ment and auricular reconstruction are combined. We generally proceed according to the following plan: a retroauricular island flap is transported forward through a tunnel created in the rudimentary auricle, which then forms the new helix. After subcutaneous removal of the available rudimen-tary cartilage, this cartilage is reimplanted at the desired site. Most patients do not wish further intervention like the insertion of costal cartilage.

With grade 3 microtia, that is, severe deformity or auricular aplasia, the question of whether an auricle ought to be constructed should first be discussed with the parents. We are all aware of how difficult it is for even an experienced plastic surgeon to achieve a reasonably good reconstruction of the auricle. The creation of attachment sites for an auricular epithesis, therefore, is often preferable, as has been shown by use of transcutaneous titanium implants anchored in the mastoid plane [Tjellström et al., 1981]. There is some hope that advances in plastic surgery are possible by subcutaneous implantation of a tissue expander.

The timing of the operative correction of the atretic canal on the opposite side should be decided on the basis of the individual patient. It depends particularly on the state of the first ear and on the changes of the second ear, for example, ventilation and size of the middle ear, as well as hearing capacity of the inner ear. Since hearing in the first ear is not complete, we prefer to do the second ear before the patient is 10 years old.

In patients with unilateral auditory canal atresia, we tend to wait until they are about 14 years old, so that the patients themselves can decide for or against surgery. At this age, the patients are usually willing and capable of cooperation, a factor which is important for the postoperative treatment. Occasionally, we also operate unilateral atresia of the auditory canal earlier if the patient expressly wishes. This depends, of course, on the anatomy of the middle ear. If computer tomography of the temporal bone does not reveal an aerated middle ear (type III cases), then surgery should not be done in unilateral cases.

The above-described procedure could only be applied in a minority of our cases, because many patients were transferred to our department at a late age (see fig. 2).

In type I cases with normal or at least fair inner ear function *explorative surgery* is often preferred to extensive radiological diagnostic procedures.

Surgical Technique

Primary reconstruction is usually performed under general anesthesia, and revision surgery in adults usually under local anesthesia. Surgery of major ear malformations is as variable as the disease itself. Nevertheless, in most patients, i.e. type II cases, we prefer the direct approach to the antrum as has been similarly used by Wigand [1978] and other authors. The technique is as follows: the approach is close to the tegmen tympani so that the facial nerve, which usually courses atypically, is not damaged. When the antrum is opened, not too wide, the body of the incus, an important landmark, should be identified which, typically, is fused with the mal-

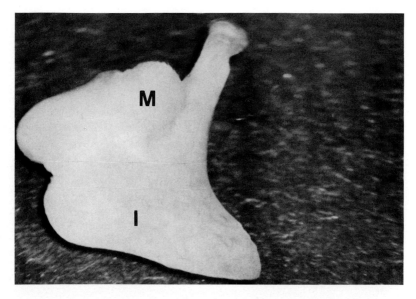

Fig. 1. Fused malleus (M) and incus (I) in a case of type II malformation. Usually the incudostapedial joint is separated and the bulky ossicular mass is removed.

leus (fig. 1). The malleus handle is most often undeveloped. It is extremely important not to touch this bony mass with the burr, and not to drill on the atretic plate before the incudostapedial joint has been separated.

The neck of the malleus, which is often attached to the bony atretic plate, is then exposed. The lamina propria of the ear drum, which is usually developed, must be preserved to ensure a favorable anterior angle. In cases where the malleus-incus mass is bulky or far under the temporomandibular joint, it should be removed, as we do nowadays in most of our type II cases in order to avoid osseous re-fixation. Then a long ceramic hollow shaft implant is fitted on the stapes head, to ensure a deep middle ear (fig. 2). Sometimes the middle ear cleft is closed by a relatively inflexible and stable disk of lyophilized dura, which is glued by tissue adhesive. More often the temporalis fascia is used and then the new auditory canal is lined with a thin Thiersch split skin graft using a modified Jahrsdoerfer technique [Jahrsdoerfer, personal commun., 1981]. Here human fibrin glue, which we otherwise use with reservation, has proved advantageous. The part of the graft covering the new tympanic membrane must be translucent as used by Belluci [1981] for his entire graft. Whenever possible the Thiersch

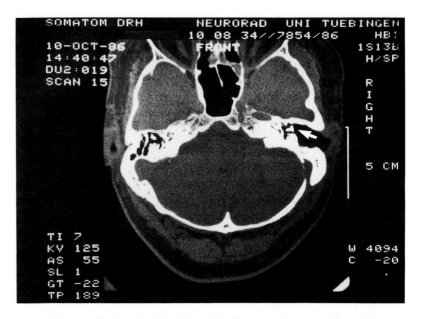

Fig. 2. CT scan of a 52-year-old patient with bilateral major ear malformation. The right ear had been previously operated on elsewhere and revised in our department. The poor pneumatization of the mastoid allowed creation of a small, self-cleaning cavity. Ossicular reconstruction was performed with a 5-mm aluminum oxide ceramic hollow-shaft implant (arrow) to the stapes head. After the CT scan was done the left auricle was reconstructed and the left ear was operated on in an analogous fashion to the right.

graft is sutured laterally in order to obtain a wide, stable entrance of the new outer auditory canal. Often the adjacent skin is sutured via burr holes in the most lateral part of the newly created bony canal walls according to Zühlke [1972]. As recently pointed out by Helms [1987] this technique prevents stenosis of the newly created external auditory canal entrance. Finally, the auditory canal is covered abundantly with silicone and packed for 3 weeks with gelfoam. In some cases – where the auricle was fairly well developed – a postauricular island flap was used to cover the new posterior canal wall and to close the opened air cell system.

The functional results achieved by this technique, which was used for 5 years, are very encouraging. In about two-thirds of the cases, the remaining air-bone gap is less than 20 dB. One important aspect is that the vibratory new ear drum plane is sufficiently large, providing, of course, that anatomic conditions were favorable. The epithelialization at the anterior parts of the new ear drum is essential. Of greatest importance is postoperative care until the ear is completely dry. A preliminary analysis of our 169 operated major ear malformation patients (1967–1986) revealed that adequate hearing was achieved in the majority of all cases; that is a conductive deficit of less than 20 dB. One-third of the patients with bilateral major ear malformations, i.e. type III cases, had fenestration of the lateral semicircular canal. This intervention made it possible for many of these patients to use a hearing aid more successfully [Plester, 1971], some had to be revised several times. Finally, it should be pointed out that revision surgery can be very worthwile. Forty-nine of our patients had previous surgery done elsewhere, some of the patients originally operated on in our department also had revision surgery, the main indications being restenosis and incomplete medial epithelialization as well as further hearing improvement. Detailed follow-up data will be published elsewhere.

References

Altmann, F.: Congenital atresia of the ear in man and animals. Ann. Otol. Rhinol. Lar. *64:* 824–858 (1955).

Belluci, R.J.: Congenital aural malformations: diagnosis and treatment. Otolar. Clins N. Am. *14:* 95–124 (1981).

Cremers, C.W.R.J.; Oudenhoven, J.M.T.M.; Marres, E.H.M.A.: Congenital aural atresia. A new subclassification and surgical management. Clin. Otolaryngol. *9:* 119–127 (1984).

de la Cruz, A.; Linthicum, F.H., Jr.; Luxford, W.M.: Congenital atresia of the external auditory canal. Laryngoscope *95:* 421–427 (1985).

Gerhardt, H.-J.: Zur Rekonstruktion von Gehörgang und Trommelfell bei kongenitaler Gehörgangsatresie. HNO Praxis *1:* 470–476 (1976).

Helms, H.: Ergebnisse der Mikrochirurgie bei Ohrmissbildungen. Lar. Rhinol. Otol. *66:* 16–18 (1987).

Jahnke, K.: Zur Chirurgie der grossen und kleinen Ohrmissbildungen. Vortrag auf der Jahrestagung des Berufsverbandes der Deutschen Hals-Nasen-Ohrenärzte, Essen 1986.

Jahrsdoerfer, R.A.: Congenital atresia of the ear. Laryngoscope *88:* suppl. 13, pp. 1–48 (1978).

Jahrsdoerfer, R.A.; Yeakley, J.W.; Hall, J.W., III; Robbins, K.T.; Gray, L.C.: High-resolution CT scanning and auditory brain stem response in congenital aural atresia. Patient selection and surgical correlation. Otolaryngol. Head Neck Surg. *93:* 292–298 (1985).

Jörgensen, G.: Missbildungen im Bereich der Hals-Nasen-Ohren-Heilkunde. Arch. klin. exp. Ohr.-Nas.-Kehlk.-Heilk. *202:* 1–50 (1972).

Marquet, J.: Homogreffes tympano-ossiculaires dans le traitement chirurgical de l'agénésie de l'oreille. Acta oto-rhino-lar. belg. *25:* 885–897 (1971).

Mündnich, K.: Operationen bei Ohrmissbildungen; in Naumann, Kopf- und Hals-Chirurgie, vol. III, pp. 383–404; 1. Aufl. (Thieme Stuttgart 1976).

Ombredanne, M.: Absence congénitale de fenêtre ronde dans certaines aplasies mineures. Annls Oto-lar. *85:* 369–378 (1968).

Ombredanne, M.: Chirurgie des surdités congénitales par malformation ossiculaires. Acta oto-rhino-lar. belg. *25:* 837–869 (1971).

Plester, D.: Congenital malformations of the middle ear. Acta oto-rhino-lar. belg. *25:* 877–884 (1971).

Schuknecht, H.F.: Reconstructive procedures for congenital aural atresia. Archs Otolar. *101:* 170–172 (1975).

Tjellström, A.; Albrektsson, T.; Lindström, J.; et al.: The bone-anchored auricular episthesis. Laryngoscope *91:* 811 (1981).

Wigand, M.E.: Tympano-méatoplastie endaurale pour les atrésies congénitales sévères de l'oreille. Revue lar. Otol. Rhinol. *99:* 15–28 (1978).

Zühlke, D.: Chirurgische Behandlung der Missbildungen des Ohres. Arch. klin. exp. Ohr.-Nas.-Kehlk.-Heilk. *202:* 153–202 (1972).

Prof. Dr. K. Jahnke, Department of Otorhinolaryngology, University of Tübingen, D–7400 Tübingen (FRG)

Adv. Oto-Rhino-Laryng., vol. 40, pp. 9–14 (Karger, Basel 1988)

Classification of Congenital Aural Atresia and Results of Reconstructive Surgery

C.W.R.J. Cremers, E. Teunissen, E.H.M.A. Marres

Department of Otorhinolaryngology, University Hospital Nijmegen, Nijmegen, The Netherlands

Introduction

Congenital aural atresia varies from a mild abnormality with narrowing of the external auditory canal and hypoplasia of the tympanic membrane and middle ear space to the entire absence of the middle ear cleft in conjunction with anotia, bony atresia of the external canal and even hypoplasia of inner ear structures.

In the early days of surgery for congenital aural atresia, failure to improve hearing, stenosis of the newly formed canal, facial nerve paralysis, discharging cavities and cosmetic disadvantages limited the rare good results. Improved microsurgical techniques, elucidation of middle ear and inner ear dynamics, understanding of tympanoplastic reconstruction and the introduction of polytomographic roentgenographic techniques and nowadays computerized axial tomography for identification of middle ear and inner ear structures are essential in the improvement of surgical results.

Altmann [1] was the first to propose an anatomical classification according to the severity of the atresia and Nager [2] and Schuknecht [3] considered his classification helpful from the surgical point of view. Nevertheless, the second class of the three classes proposed by Altmann represented the vast majority of cases. Nager [2] proposed an additional classification of the developmental anomalies of the auricle, since severe anomalies of the auricle were thought to be related to the degree of middle ear anomalies.

Additional Classification of Type II Congenital Aural Atresia

The type 1 aural atresia is presented in figure 1. The additional classification of atresia we proposed concerns type II which has to be divided in a class type IIA (fig. 2, 3) and type IIB (fig. 4). In type IIB there is a total bony stenosis over the full length of the meatus, while in type IIA (fig. 2, 3) there is a total bony atresia over only a part of the length of the meatus or the canal is partially aplastic and ends blindly with a fistula tract sometimes leading to a rudimentary tympanic membrane.

In type III aural atresia the auricle is usually severely malformed or completely absent. The external auditory canal is absent and the tympanic cavity is either very small or missing. The ossicles are rudimentary or missing and the mastoid is not pneumatized. There are frequently associated anomalies of the inner ear and severe cranial malformations. These cases are to be excluded from surgery of the middle ear. Sometimes a canal plasty procedure can be performed for rehabilitation with a hearing aid in the rare case the auricle is so well developed that a hearing aid can be adapted. This additional subclassification for congenital aural atresia type II has been published previously [4–7].

General Management and Preoperative Evaluation

The main purpose of surgery is to give the patient serviceable hearing, corresponding to an average hearing threshold level below 30–35 dB ISO for 0.5 and 2 kHz. In cases of unilateral atresia it can result in binaural hearing, with the best results when the hearing level approaches that of the other ear.

In our opinion prerequisites for surgery are: (1) normal cochlear function in the ear to be operated upon; (2) polytomography or CT scan to show an ossicular chain and a clearly well-developed middle ear cavity; (3) some pneumatization of the mastoid, and (4) in unilateral cases a cosmetic appearance of the auricle that can be accepted as a good end result with or without cosmetic surgery.

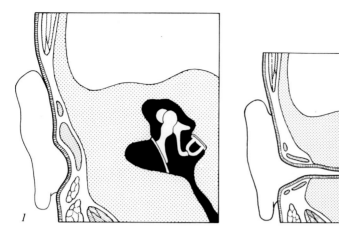

Fig. 1. Type I congenital aural atresia (according to Altmann [1]), with an intact tympanic membrane and bony atresia of the lateral part of the external auditory canal.

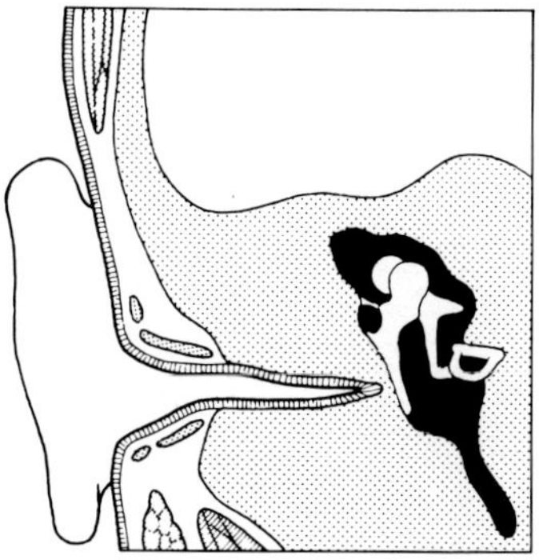

Fig. 2. A type IIA congenital aural atresia with a fistula tract ending blindly.

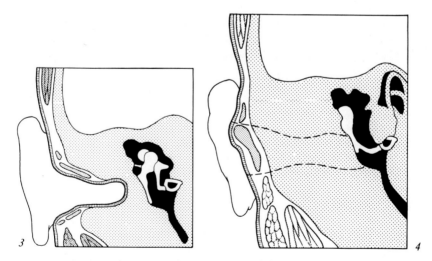

Fig. 3. A type IIA congenital aural atresia with a total bony atresia over only a part of the canal.

Fig. 4. Type IIB congenital aural atresia.

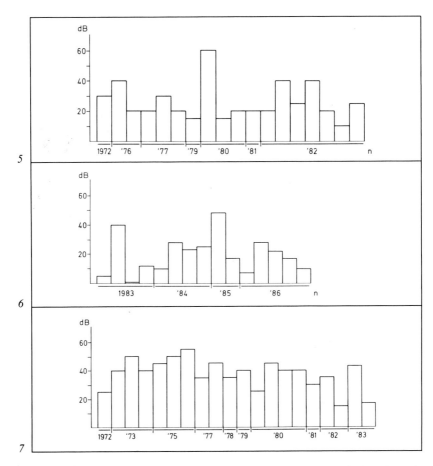

Fig. 5. Postoperative air-bone gap in 18 ears with a type IIA congenital aural atresia over the period 1972–1982.

Fig. 6. Postoperative air-bone gap in 15 ears with a type IIA congenital aural atresia over the period 1983–1986.

Fig. 7. Postoperative air-bone gap in 20 ears with a type IIB congenital aural atresia over the period 1972–1986.

Surgical Technique, Patients and Results

Nowadays fenestration of the lateral semicircular canal has been abandoned as method of choice for surgery of congenital aural atresia. Currently used methods are the type III tympanoplasty [3], the canal plasty [4]

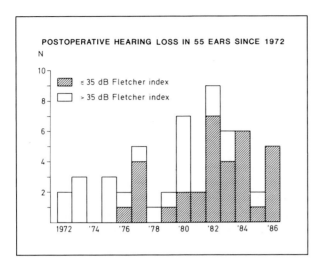

Fig. 8. Postoperative hearing loss in 55 ears with a type I, IIA or IIB congenital aural atresia, since 1972.

and the canal plasty with allograft tympanoplasty. The canal plasty procedure we use has been described previously [5]. The results obtained in the first 36 ears with a type II atresia over the period 1972–1983 have been reported [4–6].

Of 55 ears of 48 patients with a type I or II anomaly, operated upon in the Nijmegen Department of Otorhinolaryngology over the period 1972–1986, 2 ears had a type I anomaly, 33 a type IIA and 20 a type IIB anomaly. The average preoperative threshold for the speech frequencies 0.5, 1 and 2 kHz was 44 dB (range 38–50 dB) in group I, 47 dB (range 25–77 dB) in group IIA, and 58 dB (range 30–70 dB) in group IIB atresia. The postoperative average threshold was 21 dB (range 20–22 dB) in group I, 26 dB (range 10–60 dB) in group IIA, and 38 dB (range 15–55 dB) in group IIB.

Detailed postoperative results are presented separately for class IIA (fig. 5, 6) and class IIB (fig. 7). The average hearing gain was 21 dB for group IIA and 20 dB for group IIB. An overview of the 55 ears with a type I, IIA and IIB classification operated on from 1972 to 1986 with a postoperative hearing loss of 35 dB or less or larger then 35 dB Fletcher Index is shown in figure 8.

Postoperative complications of this surgery can be sensorineural deafness, facial paralysis, perforation of the tympanic membrane, restenosis and otorrhea. None of these patients had a sensorineural hearing loss or facial paralysis following surgery.

In some patients with bilateral atresia a sensorineural component was only recognized in the audiogram after previous surgery elsewhere and our end results were therefore restricted. A perforation of the tympanic membrane occurred only twice. A total restenosis was seen in 4 patients and in 9 treatment was given for long-standing otorrhea, leading to dry ears in 8 of them. In the last 3 years we have not had any of these side effects.

Comment

Additional classification and strict criteria for surgery, such as age and the absence of a sensorineural component in the hearing loss are required to select the successful cases preoperatively. This improved our rate of success to such an extent that a small group of patients with unilateral atresia has also had benefit from surgery in recent years. Since the group of unilateral atresia is 4–5 times as frequent as the bilateral group, this has opened possibilities for a large number of patients with unilateral aural atresia, type IIA. Possibly, this can also be expanded to type IIB unilateral atresia since the surgical experience may improve yet further.

References

1   Altmann, F.: Congenital aural atresia of the ear in man and animals. Ann. Otol. Rhinol. Lar. *64:* 824–858 (1955).
2   Nager, G.T.: Congenital aural atresia. Anatomy and surgical management. Birth Defects *4:* 33–51 (1971).
3   Schuknecht, H.F.: Reconstructive procedures for congenital aural atresia. Archs Otolar. *101:* 170–172 (1975).
4   Cremers, C.W.R.J.; Oudenhoven, J.M.T.M.; Marres, F.H.M.A.: Congenital aural atresia. A new subclassification and surgical management. Clin. Otolar. *9:* 119–127 (1984).
5   Marres, E.H.M.A.; Cremers, C.W.R.J.: Surgical treatment of congenital aural atresia. Am. J. Otol. *6:* 247–249 (1985).
6   Cremers, C.W.R.J.; Marres, E.H.M.A.: An additional classification for congenital aural atresia. Its impact on the predictability of surgical results. Acta oto-rhino-lar. belg. (in press, 1986).
7   Cremers, C.W.R.J.: Surgery in congenital aural atresia (Editorial). Clin. Otolar. *10:* 61–62 (1985).

C.W.R.J. Cremers, MD, Department of Otorhinolaryngology,
University Hospital Nijmegen, NL–6500 HD Nijmegen (The Netherlands)

Adv. Oto-Rhino-Laryng., vol. 40, pp. 15–23 (Karger, Basel 1988)

Allografts and Congenital Aural Atresia

J. Marquet [1]

ENT Department, University of Antwerp, Antwerp, Belgium

Introduction

The surgical treatment of congenital malformations of the ear, and more particularly congenital aural atresia, has to be considered as one of the most difficult tasks facing the otologist. A precise preoperative assessment is always indispensable and should include audiological, radiological, psychological and mental evaluations.

After a brief review of minor anomalies, this paper is devoted to the surgical treatment of congenital ear atresia. The problems of congenital atretic ears are related to the degree reached in normal development of the lateral pharyngeal groove in the first instance and secondly the degree of differentiation of the tympanic ring. Consequently, there are two basic types of atresia. In the first the morphological differentiation of the lateral pharyngeal groove is normal or nearly so, and the problems of atresia mainly are related to the failure of full differentiation of the tympanic bone and the formation of the external auditory canal. As a result the facial nerve follows its normal course and the middle ear anomalies of the ossicular chain are minimal, whereas the external auditory canal is occluded in its medial two-thirds by fibrous tissue or bone. Usually, the characteristic space between the posterior wall of the glenoid cavity and the anterior wall of the mastoid not only exists but has the same dimensions as those of the fully differentiated normal ear.

[1] With thanks to Mr. J.D.K. Dawes, who kindly helped to edit this paper in English.

In the second type of major atresia the lateral pharyngeal groove is less well differentiated and the dysmorphia in the middle ear structures is usually worse: The 'characteristic space' in the neighbourhood of the mandibular joint is absent and the facial nerve nearly always follows an abnormal course. The appearances suggest that the region of the whole external auditory meatus is missing.

While the minor malformations generally associated with a normal external auditory canal are amenable to the classic functional middle ear surgical approaches, major malformations combined with external canal or pinnal deformities require a more complex and carefully planned surgical approach. Various techniques have been proposed, each with its own advantages and disadvantages. These various techniques are not discussed in this paper, which is devoted entirely to the technique which we have used for more than 25 years. This technique has also been published elsewhere [6].

Where possible an open cavity should be avoided. To this end, a mastoid opening is created as far posteriorly as possible so that the depth of the mastoid may be gauged, the lateral semicircular canal and the short process of the incus identified. Then a new external auditory canal can be created leaving a bony posterior wall between the canal and the cavity. The equivalent of a posterior tympanotomy view of the middle ear can be obtained, and the result similar to the combined approach tympanoplasty or 'intact wall' mastoidectomy.

The ossicles are always treated conservatively for they are frequently functional and useful in reconstruction. In reconstruction preference is given to the use of 'tympanomeatal' allografts. These grafts consist of the fibrous part of the external auditory canal and tympanic membrane with an intact annulus and where necessary the attached ossicular chain. The allografts are preserved according to the method described by Marquet [1–6]. The chosen graft is used as a model for sculpturing a new bony external auditory canal and bony sulcus for the annulus. As a one-stage operation this technique gives valuable functional results, a safe anatomical restoration of the external auditory canal, and very acceptable esthetic results depending of course on the severity of the anomalies found. Postoperative stenosis is exceptional, and infections are rare. No rejection phenomena have been encountered so far. A follow-up of more than 25 years has shown that the results obtained may be considered definitive and that this technique seems to be the safest available.

Surgical Techniques

Preoperative Evaluation

The main goals of this type of surgery are: (1) overall improvement in hearing; (2) minimization of the risks of postoperative complications, and (3) improvement in cosmetic appearance.

Audiology

A preliminary examination is carried out with great care to exclude any sensorineural deafness which is of a severity that would make surgery useless. Even using all the facilities offered by modern audiology this evaluation can sometimes be difficult, especially when the patient has a psychological disorder.

Radiology

Plain radiographs tomograms or CT scan are the most important preoperative investigations, and should never be omitted. The surgeon needs to know the type of malformation before surgery, and whether or not the lesion is too extensive for surgical treatment.

Psychosocial Evaluation

These considerations may also influence the decision to operate for some social situations or psychological disorders are incompatible with the required postoperative care or follow-up. The cooperation of a psychiatrist, pediatrician and psychologist is always useful, and at times indispensable.

Age of the Patient

The average age suitable for this type of surgery is between 6 and 12 years of age. Most authors agree that surgery must never be carried out before 5 years of age. In our opinion, even in bilateral cases operation before this age is never indicated, because audiophonetic effects of the conductive type of deafness can always be controlled by the use of a hearing aid. An operation carried out at an earlier age rarely produces good functional results.

Unilateral Malformations

The dispute about surgery on unilateral severe malformations still continues. Most authors agree that surgery should never be proposed for unilateral disease. We believe that this attitude is conditioned by the present high rate of complications and the often poor functional long-term results. The use of allograft tympanic membrane and external auditory canal skin, which gives good anatomical results, has led us to change our policy. At present we advocate surgery for unilateral anomalies, provided that the pre-operative assessment suggests a good prognosis.

Cosmetic Surgery

The new external auditory canal must be rebuilt in functional continuity with the middle ear cavity and ossicular chain. The canal must be reconstituted before any cosmetic surgery is carried out. Plastic surgery on the pinna is only acceptable if it is centred on the new meatus at the first operation or as a second stage operation. It must never be done before the anatomical and functional reconstruction of the meatus and middle ear.

Surgical Treatment

General Principles

Many complications can be avoided if certain principles are kept in mind. If there is bony fixation of the ossicular chain, and in particular of the handle of the malleus, to the tympanic ring, drilling or the use of the cutting burr should be used as little as possible in order to avoid the risk of sensorineural deafness due to acoustic trauma. The noise produced by such drilling is between 160 and 200 dB. Curettes should therefore be used to remove the bone remnants around the ossicles. A full-thickness skin graft is taken preferably from the retroauricular area of the neck which is hairless, for permanent hair growth in a new auditory canal is always troublesome. Large cavities which include the mastoid cells can cause persistent mucous or mucopurulent discharge from the ear, these ears are always difficult to dry up and so open cavities should be avoided. In order to preserve the surgical field for possible later cosmetic surgery the incisions must be reduced to a minimum and the underlying tissues always respected. Scar tissue around the pinna, resulting from too extensive a dissection or too large an incision, creates problems for plastic reconstruction of the pinna.

Surgical Technique

The main features of our surgical technique are based upon the use of a tympanomeatal or monobloc allograft and we regard congenital aural atresia as one of the main indications for its use. In a one-stage procedure it is possible to produce a safe anatomical reconstruction of the external auditory canal, valuable functional hearing improvement and very acceptable esthetic appearance.

The main points of this technique are:

Incision. An incision is started at the level of the superior edge of the pinna and extended posteriorly and inferiorly along the hairline to the insertion of the sternomastoid. The incision can be extended further into the neck. This provides a large retroauricular area as a donor site for a free full-thickness skin graft which can be of varied length and width and is usually made spear shaped as this shape is most useful for the restoration of the lateral part of the external auditory meatus. The skin is elevated anteriorly to uncover the posterior wall of the glenoid cavity and an incision is made through the periosteum around the glenoid cavity and then elevated posteriorly as an intact periosteal layer to form a covering for the new external meatus.

Bony Exposure. The zona cribrosa and linea temporalis are identified and, using these surface landmarks as a guide, the mastoid is gently drilled to expose the middle fossa dura superiorly and the sigmoid sinus posteriorly. The mastoid cells are opened and a triangular cavity created as far posteriorly as possible. The depth of the mastoid can now be assessed and the short process of the incus identified. Once this identification has been made, the new external auditory canal can be created, great care being taken as the canal is deepened to avoid damage to the ossicular chain. The excavation of the mastoid and ear canal created conditions similar to those of the combined approach tympanoplasty.

Reconstruction of the Ossicular Chain and Tympanic Membrane. The middle ear cavity is thoroughly inspected and the ossicular chain although deformed and fixed is carefully freed and, if still functional, preserved. Otherwise an ossiculoplasty is performed. Care must be taken not to displace the ossicular chain with a drill to avoid acoustic trauma. A bony annulus is then rebuilt using a cutting burr and the external auditory canal shaped to put the tympano-meatal allograft or monobloc so that the annulus and tympanic membrane will get snugly into position and in perfect contact with the ossicular chain (fig. 1).

Three of four holes are drilled in the lateral wall of the newly created external canal so that 000 nylon threads will pass through to fix the allograft and skin graft closely adjacent to each other. A vertical incision is then made behind the tragus of the deformed pinna and the posterior and superior parts of the pinna are retracted upwards and backwards to obtain a normal curve to the new meatal entrance. The full-thickness graft is then sutured helicoidally into the lateral part of the external canal lying against the cuff of the allograft on its medial surface and being sutured to the edges of the pinnal opening (fig. 2).

The end result is to procure satisfactory continuity between the original skin of the pinna anterior and posterior to the new external auditory canal and the allograft skin. Furthermore, the posterosuperior retraction of the pinna obtained by suturing of the postaural wound produces a satisfactory esthetic effect. The new external auditory canal is packed with artificial sponges which are left in place for 8 days (fig. 3).

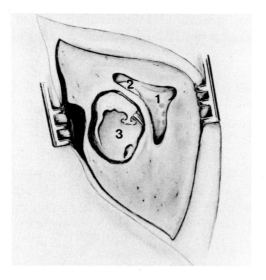

Fig. 1. 1 = Mastoidectomy; 2 = lateral semicircular canal; 3 = new external auditory canal.

This technique provides a satisfactory restoration of the external auditory canal, an overgrowth of new skin layer around the canal itself, and the placement of a natural physiological eardrum on top of a functional ossicular chain. So far, rejection has not occurred.

Associated Anomalies

One cannot study malformations of the middle ear without considering the associated problems often caused by the facial nerve, malformations of the pinna, the often associated fistula, and congenital cholesteatoma.

Facial Nerve

The facial nerve, which is the branchial nerve of the second or hyoid branchial arch, is associated with a great number of the 'malformations'. In the tympanic segment of the Fallopian canal the most frequent anomaly is *dehiscence* of its *bony covering.*

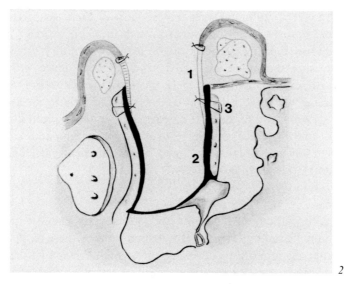

2

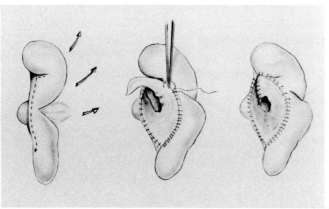

3

Fig. 2. 1 = Full-thickness autograft; 2 = tympano-meatal allograft; 3 = nylon threads.

Fig. 3. Reconstruction of the new meatal entrance.

Duplication, reduplication and triplication of the nerve have been described. An abnormal course has also been observed. The nerve or the duplicated neural fibres pass through the arch of the stapes. In the mastoid segment a pronounced posterior displacement has been reported; other cases have also been described with courses not only posteriorly but also laterally. More severe anomalies such as hypoplasia or even agenesis of the facial nerve are unfortunately sometimes present in severe atresia.

In the case of type IV agenesis of the external auditory canal [6], unusual courses of the nerve are well known. In accordance with the embryological description of this anomaly, the nerve turns anteriorly at the level of the round window, instead of continuing inferiorly to the anteriorly situated stylomastoid foramen. This particular anomaly prohibits any drilling work inferiorly and anteriorly to enlarge the tympanic cavity. These anomalies of the facial nerve have been studied in particular by Miehlke [7] and Crabtree [8].

The Pinna

Major malformations of the pinna are generally associated with the middle ear anomalies and vice versa. However, a series of these malformations shows that the amount of development or maldevelopment has no direct relationship to the degree of deformity of the middle ear cleft. A wide range of anomalies of the pinna have been described from the minor architectural anomalies to the total absence of the pinna, named according to the embryological development pattern – dysmorphic auricles, accessory auricles, or the most common 'the question mark pinna'. In the majority of cases the outline of the tragus remains, which is very important from the cosmetic point of view.

Congenital Aural Fistula

The most frequent fistulae are located anterior to the pinna and are generally associated with minor ossicular anomalies. Cysts or fistulae originating from the first or the second branchial grooves are rare. Those arising from the first branchial grooves are situated between the lobe of the ear and the inferior part of the external auditory canal, and may pass through the parotid gland. Those arising from the second branchial groove are more characteristic; the external orifice is situated anterior to the sternomastoid muscle, while the medial end lies in the middle ear cleft.

Cholesteatoma

The existence of congenital cholesteatoma has been proved by surgical findings. The disease is more frequent in terotological embryopathies, especially when there is a severe congenital atresia, as with thalidomide which has been responsible for the most severe ear malformations and fetal damage ever seen.

Conclusion

Surgery for congenital middle ear malformations by using allograft material provides very satisfactory results from both the functional and anatomical points of view. Nevertheless, it must not be forgotten that one of the most important parts of this surgical work concerns the evaluation of each case and assessing its prognosis. Any kind of surgical adventure should be avoided. This implies that this type of surgery must be reserved for well-trained surgeons. Above all, the principle, 'primum non nocere' should be kept in mind.

References

1   Marquet, J.F.: Proceedings of the International Congress of Otolaryngology, Mexico vol. 206, pp. 151–159 (Excerpta Medica, Amsterdam 1969).
2   Marquet, J.F.: Considérations sur le diagnostic des surdités de transmission par traumatisme de l'oreille. Acta oto-rhino-lar. belg. *25:* 641–652 (1971).
3   Marquet, J.F.: Homogreffes tympano-ossiculaires dans le traitement chirurgical de l'agénésie de l'oreille. Acta oto-rhino-lar. belg. *25:* 885–897 (1971).
4   Marquet, J.F.: Current status of tympanic membrane implants. Fifth International Workshop on Middle Ear Microsurgery and Fluctuant Hearing Loss, Chicago 1976 (Strode, Huntsville 1976).
5   Marquet, J.F.: Twelve years' experience with homograft tympanoplasty. Otolar. Clins N. Am. *10:* 581–593 (1977).
6   Marquet, J.F.: Congenital conductive deafness; in Maran, Stell, Clinical otolaryngology, pp. 501–513 (Blackwell, Oxford 1979).
7   Miehlke, A.: Surgery of the facial nerve; 2nd ed., pp. 9–21 (Urban & Schwarzenberg, München 1973).
8   Crabtree, J.A.: The facial nerve in congenital ear surgery. Otolar. Clins N. Am. *7:* 505 (1974).

J. Marquet, MD, Fruithoflaan 91/12, B–2600 Berchem (Belgium)

Adv. Oto-Rhino-Laryng., vol. 40, pp. 24–32 (Karger, Basel 1988)

Use of Tissue Integrated Implants in Congenital Aural Malformations

A. Tjellström[a], *M. Jacobsson*[a], *T. Albrektsson*[b], *K. Jansson*[a]

[a] ENT Department Sahlgrenska sjukhuset, and
[b] Department of Handicap Research, University of Göteborg, Göteborg, Sweden

Introduction

According to the Swedish Board of Welfare statistics the frequency of isolated external ear and external ear canal malformations in 1980 amounted to 0.92 per 10,000 live births. If live-born children with other defects such as Treacher Collins and similar syndroms were included, the yearly incidence of congenital aural defects was found to be 0.4% [Lidén et al., 1983]. In the city of Göteborg 57,172 live births were registered between 1970 and 1979 [Kankkunen, 1982]. Among these children 120 were diagnosed as hard of hearing or deaf due to congenital defects. This means a prevalence of 0.21%. The number of external ear and/or external ear canal defects among these 120 children were 23 or 19.1%. The frequency of these types of defects among these live born children in Göteborg 1970–1979 could thus be calculated to be 3.6 per 10,000. Fairly great variations in the incidence between different years have been found and the causes for these variations have been discussed by Lidén et al. [1983] but not always have there been clear causes of these discrepancies. If, however, the figures presented here are used, the total number of individuals with an external ear and/or external ear canal abnormality in Sweden, with 8 million inhabitants, could be estimated to be around 3,000. Even if all of these are not suitable for reconstructive surgery there will still be a large number of patients that would have an increased quality of life with an external ear. At the American Academy meeting in Atlanta 1985 Dr. James Crabtree stated in his Instructional Course on Management of Congenital Aural Atresia that 'this type of surgery could be considered as one of the most difficult ones in otology'. At the ENT Department, Sahlgren's Hospital, University of Göteborg, Sweden, we have for many years taken a conservative attitude to atresia operations with the objective to improve hearing. Thus, we consider surgery on unilateral congenital atresia as almost contraindicated. This attitude has also been advocated by several leading otologists in the USA [Hough, personal commun., 1983]. In our department we have taken almost the same conservative attitude towards bilateral atresia as our experience with hearing through direct bone conduction with the bone-anchored hearing aid (BAHA) has grown. Reconstructive surgery to establish an external ear, in cases of rudimentary external ear rests, has also been abandoned by many otologists [Tjellström et al., 1985]. A prosthetic device often gives a much better cosmetic result and the surgical procedures are much more simple. The lower costs for the patient/insurance company/society should be taken into consideration.

Aim of the Study

The aim of this presentation is to briefly present the surgical concept for retention of the prosthesis on tissue integrated implants, in some detail explain how the prosthesis is made and finally present our experience with this type of silicon rubber prosthesis in children.

Methods and Materials

Surgical Technique

The surgical technique has been described in detail by Tjellström [1985] and only a short summary will be presented. It is a two-stage procedure with 3–4 months in between the operations. The procedures are generally made under local anaesthesia and takes about 45 min. At the first stage operation three to four implants made out of commercially pure titanium are placed in the temporal bone with a well defined surgical technique. The screw shaped implants, the fixtures, are 3.75 mm in diameter and come in two standard lengths, 3.0 and 4.0 mm (fig. 1). At the second stage operation the skin-penetrating titanium abutments are attached to the fixtures. These abutments will provide retention for the prosthesis.

Manufacturing of the Prosthesis

The first step is to take an impression of the abutments and the surrounding area. If there is an external ear canal opening this is packed with gauze in order to prevent foreign ingress of material. Specially shaped impression copings with long guide pins are attached

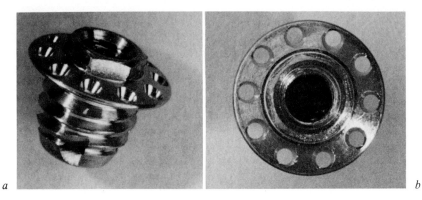

a *b*

Fig. 1. Flange fixture of commercially pure titanium used for retention of auricular prostheses.

to the percutaneous abutment. Dental floss is wound around and between the impression copings. The floss is then covered with self-curing acrylic. A special cylindrical impression tray made of boxing wax is placed around the prepared area (fig. 2a). A low viscosity alginate mixture is used to make the impression. When the alginate has set, the top of the box is filled with quick-set plaster (fig. 2b). When the plaster material has set, the guide pins are unscrewed and the impression is carefully removed. Brass replicas are then attached to the impression coping. The impression with the copings and replicas is now poured in an improved dental stone. When the impression is separated from the cast an exact working model of the patient's defect area has been created with the brass replicas on exactly the same spot, direction and height as the skin-penetrating abutments (fig. 2c, d). In order to facilitate the sculpturing of an auricular prosthesis, an impression of the opposite ear is made. This impression is poured in plaster and used during sculpturing of the prosthetic ear. Gold caps are then attached to the brass replicas of the working model (fig. 2e). A gold bar is fitted to the grooves in the gold caps. The bar should be extended 10–15 mm beyond the terminal abutment in order to facilitate retention of the prosthesis. The bar is temporarily attached to the gold caps with soldering wax (fig. 2f). The construction is removed from the working model and soldered. Following soldering, the bar construction is carefully checked on the working cast and on the patient. Adjustments are made if necessary. When the bar construction fits perfectly, it is placed on the working model and retention elements (Öquist clips) are positioned on the bar, undercuts are blocked out with wax and autopolymerizing acrylic resin is poured over the bar clip apparatus. The acrylic resin plate is tried on the patient to verify fit and contours (fig. 2g). The wax ear is then placed on the plate on the patient in order to identify the correct orientation and verify contours. Care is taken that the abutments are not totally sealed from the outside of the model. Air must have access to the skin to prevent irritation due to moisture accumulation. When the wax ear model and the acrylic resin plate demonstrate optimal fit, they are embedded in a mould of plaster consisting of three parts (fig. 2h). The wax is then removed with hot water (fig. 2i).

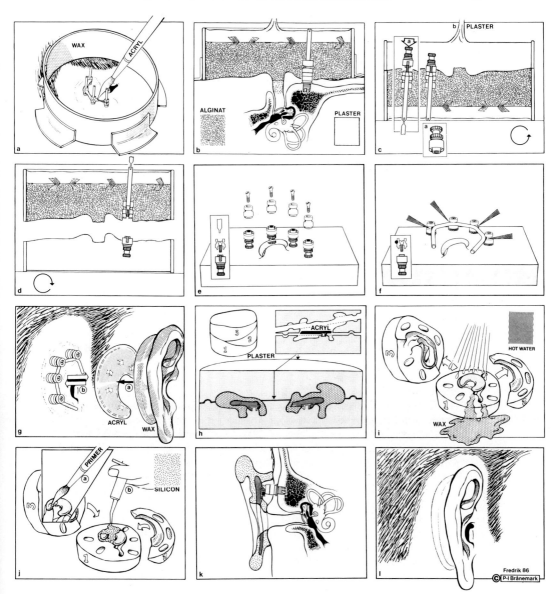

Fig. 2. Illustration of some of the steps at the manufacturing of the auricular prosthesis. For details see text.

Table I. Patient material

Patient No.	Sex	Age of fixture operation (years/months)	Number of fixtures inserted	Follow-up time from fixture insertion (years/months)
1	M	6/7	3	1/11
2	F	9/6	3	9 months
3	F	11 years	4	4/4
4	M	9/8	4	3/9
5	M	9/8	4	3/9
6	F	11/7	4	4/6
7	M	11/1	2	1/1
8	F	9/11	3	2/9
Totals		9/11	27	x = 2/10

An important part of the procedure is the preparation of the acrylic plate for bonding of the silicone. After this, the acrylic plate is placed in the mould. The silicone is mixed to resemble the skin colour of the patient as closely as possible and is then placed in the mould (fig. 2j). When the silicone has polymerized, the prosthesis is carefully removed and adjusted as needed. Extrinsic colour arts are applied (fig. 2k). The prosthesis is then delivered to the patient (fig. 2l).

Patient Material

The first patient to receive an auricular prothesis retained on tissue integrated implants was operated upon in 1979. This was an elderly man, who had lost his external ear due to tumour surgery. Until December 21, 1986, 68 patients had been operated upon and 8 out of these were below the age of 12 at the time of the first stage operation. Four of these patients were girls and 4 were boys. All these were children with congenital defects. The oldest child in this group was 11 years and 7 months and the youngest 6 years and 7 months. The mean age was 9 years 11 months (table I). Our routine has been to use four mm long implants if sufficient thickness of the bone in the area was available, otherwise a three mm long fixture has been used. Twenty seven implants were installed, half of which were 4 mm, and half 3 mm long. According to the surgical notes three of the implants were in touch with the dura surface but the wall of the sigmoid sinus could not be seen in the bottom of any of the prepared holes. The air cells of the mastoid were entered 4 times and in 5 instances the bone available was less than 2.0 mm thick. However, all children who were taken to surgery got at least two fixtures. The surgery, as well as the healing period was uneventful in all children and the second stage operation was performed 4–14 months after the first one. Three to four weeks were allowed for healing after the second stage operation before the work on the prosthesis was started. During the first week after the impression had been taken, a working plaster model was made, and the bar for the retention was constructed. This lab period was followed by a 3-day working period on the child, when an impression of the normal ear was taken, a wax model made and the silicon

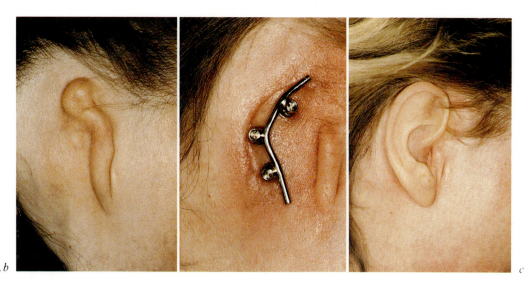

a, b   *c*

Fig. 3. Girl with a congenital malformation who at the age of 11 years and 7 months got implants for retention of an auricular prosthesis. *a* Preoperative situation. *b* Three percutaneous abutments and the bar construction. *c* The silicon rubber prosthesis in place.

Table II. Staging of skin reactions

0	No adverse skin reaction
1	Slight redness, temporary treatment with ointment (Terracortril with Polymyxin B®) for 2–3 days
2	Red and slightly moist tissue; no granuloma formation; local treatment as above, but extended; extra control visits arranged
3	Reddish and moist; sometimes granulation tissue; local revision of the affected area and granulation tissue, if present, is performed
4	Removal of skin-penetrating implant necessary due to infection
5	Removal implant for reasons not related to skin problems

rubber prosthesis casted. After a final adjustment of shape and colour the prosthesis was given to the patients.

In figure 3 a child with an auricular prosthesis retained on tissue integrated implant is shown.

Results

The first follow-up visit after the prosthesis had been given to the patient was usually after 3–5 weeks. At this visit minor adjustments of the prosthesis were made and the status of the skin around the skin-penetrating abutments was checked and recorded. The patients and their parents were instructed to keep the area clean with soap and water and once or twice a week for the first months to use ointment (Terracortril with Polymyxin B, Pfizer Inc.). The children were also instructed not to use the prosthesis during sleep in order to ensure adequate areation of the skin. The patients were then again checked 3 months after the second stage-operation and then at 6-month intervals. At these specific times the reaction of the skin around the skin-penetrating abutments were graded according to the standard presented by Holgers et al. [1986] and presented in table II. In figure 4 and table III the findings among the children in this study are presented. Out of the 95 observations judged as grade 0, one girl (patient No. 6) in spite of this lack of adverse skin reaction experienced pain and the implant was found not to be integrated. This was noted already at the second stage procedure but an abutment was attached in spite of this. After removal, which took place 3 months after the second stage operation, the pain disappeared. In analyzing the 18 situations where

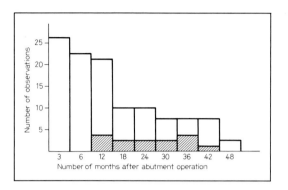

Fig. 4. Skin reactions. Total number of observations = 113. ☐ = No adverse skin reaction = 95; ▨ = adverse skin reaction = 18. Extraction of implants due to nonintegration = 1 (after 6 months in patient No. 6).

skin reaction 1 or 2 were noted all, but one, of these reactions were observed in 2 of the girls, who were also the oldest ones among the children. The problems started when they reached the age of 14 and 15, respectively, and both had a quite difficult adolescence and did not allow their parents to keep the peri-abutment areas clean. One of these girls used her prosthesis for 3 weeks without removing it even at night.

Discussion

Tissue-integrated titanium implants with percutaneous connections have been used in our department for 10 years. In children it has been used for 5 years. No major complications have been registered. The technique has been used for retention of bone conduction hearing aids as well as for craniofacial prostheses. The importance of having external ears for a young person, especially when approaching adolescence has appeared to be much greater than we first anticipated. The youngest child we have in our group was 6 years and 7 months. This is an age when a child starts to become more and more aware of physical defects and there is a risk of the child becoming subjected to, for example, teasing at school. The psychological effect of an auricular prosthesis has also been found to be surprisingly high even when the child has had other defects that may seem to be much more obvious than the external ear defect, for example in children with Treacher

Table III.

Patient No.	Number of abutments	Grading of skin reaction, months after abutment operation								
		3	6	12	18	24	30	36	42	48
1	3	0	0	0						
		0	0	0						
		0	0	0						
2	3	0								
		0								
		0								
3	4	0	0	0	0	0	0	2	0	
		0	0	0	0	0	0	2	0	
		0	0	0	0	0	0	2	0	
		0	0	0	0	0	0	2	0	
4	4	0	0	1						
		0	0	0						
		0	0	0						
		0	0	0						
5	3	0	0	0						
		0	0	0						
		0	0	0						
6	4	0	0							
		0	0	1	2	2	1	0	0	0
		0	0	1	2	2	1	0	0	0
		0	0	1	2	2	1	0	1	0
7	2	0	0							
		0	0							
8	3	0	0	0	0	0				
		0	0	0	0	0				
		0	0	0	0	0				

Collins syndrome. The possibility to have the hair styled more freely has been pointed out by several of the children and their parents as one significant advantage and giving a feeling of higher self esteem.

In the adult patients we have experienced problems around the skin-penetration among patients with psychological disturbances such as mental retardation, drug and alcohol abuse. We also noted that some patients having problems with their percutaneous abutments had a very poor personal hygiene, and in those cases, where this could be improved, the problems were often solved. It should be noted, in this respect, that it was the two girls in their puberty who had problems. To have a good personal contact with the patients and their parents is of utmost importance to avoid adverse tissue reactions. This can sometimes be difficult to predict as many of these families have been influenced deeply by their situation and an aggressive attitude is not uncommon. In some cases a postponement of surgery until the social situation has been stabilized can be necessary. On the other hand, a well-functioning prosthesis could, as mentioned above, improve the general attitude and help the child pass this difficult part in his/her life.

References

Crabtree, J.: Management of congenital aural atresia. Ann. Meet. Am. Acad. Otolaryngology – Head and Neck Surgery Course No. 2416, Atlanta 1985.
Holgers, K.-M.; Tjellström, A.; Bjursten, L.-M.; Erlandsson, B.E.: Soft tissue reactions around percutaneous implants. A preliminary report. Am. J. Otol. (accepted for publication, 1986).
Kankkunen, A.; Lidén, G.: Early identification of hearing handicapped children. Acta oto-lar., suppl. 386 (1982).
Lidén, G.; Kankkunen, A.; Tjellström, A.: Multiple handicaps and ear malformations in hearing impaired preschool children; in Mencher, Gerber, The multiply handicapped hearing impaired child, p. 67 (Grune & Stratton, New York 1983).
Tjellström, A.: Percutaneous implants in clinical practice. CRC crit. Rev. Biocompat. *I:* 205 (1985).
Tjellström, A.; Yontachev, E.; Lindström, J.; Brånemark, P.-I.: Five years experience with bone-anchored auricular protheses. Otolar. Head Neck Surg. *93:* 366 (1985).

A. Tjellström, MD, PhD, ENT Department, Sahlgrenska sjukhuset,
University of Göteborg, S–413 45 Göteborg (Sweden)

Adv. Oto-Rhino-Laryng., vol. 40, pp. 33–37 (Karger, Basel 1988)

Surgical Management of Congenital Absence of the Oval Window with Malposition of the Facial Nerve

Jean-Marc Sterkers[a], *Olivier Sterkers*[b]

[a] Service d'ORL Pédiatrique, Hôpital St-Vincent-de-Paul, Paris, France;
[b] Service d'ORL, Hôpital Beaujon, Clichy, France

Introduction

Congenital anomaly of the ossicular chain or oval window is suggested by a nonprogressive, marked, conductive hearing loss, either unilateral or bilateral, dating from birth or early childhood. Among these congenital anomalies are fixation of the footplate, nonunion of the incus and stapes, absence of the incus, and absence of the oval window [5, 6, 9]. This last anomaly is an extremely uncommon defect, since before 1958 no case could be found in the literature [5], and since then no more than 20 cases were reported [1, 3–11, 13]. The absence of the oval window is generally associated with an abnormal course of the facial nerve, and the malposition of the facial nerve over the oval window niche is thought to prevent the formation of the footplate [2].

We report hercin 4 bilateral cases in two members of two families. The 2 first cases observed in a family have been described previously in detail [11]. The conductive deafness was corrected surgically in 6 out of 8 cases. Surgical management have consisted in the insertion of a piston through a fenestra which was drilled into the vestibule just above the malpositioned facial nerve.

Material and Methods

Bilateral severe conductive deafness was found in a brother and a sister of two families, a caucasian and a black family. Anomaly of the external ear (bifid tragus) was observed in only one case. In each family, the parents were free of the disease. Children

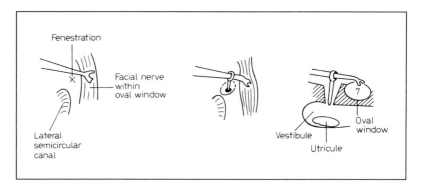

Fig. 1. Schematic drawing of the congenital defect (left panel) and of the surgical procedure utilized (middle and right panels) in all the cases.

were operated on from 4 to 8 years old. In all the cases, a similar surgical procedure was used. The middle ear was explored through a transmeatal route, and the following anomalies were found (fig. 1): (i) no facial canal in its tympanic segment; (ii) uncovered facial nerve crossed the oval window fossa; (iii) no footplate in the oval window fossa; (iv) abnormal short and thin incus; (v) rudimentary stapes with a small head and two short crura; (vi) unfixed malleus and incus, except in two ears from two different children. No other anomaly was observed, and specially the chorda tympani and the round window were present. As shown in figure 1, a fenestra was drilled above the facial nerve at the usual place of the Fallopian canal, just anterior to the ampulla of the lateral semicircular canal. When the labyrinth was opened, a Teflon piston of either 0.6 or 0.4 mm was inserted in the vestibular cavity and hung to the long process of the incus. In some cases, the incus was so thin that the piston was maintained by the addition of a small piece of bone in the piston ring. Fat and clots were placed around the piston. The perilymphatic pressure was normal.

In two ears from two different children, the malleus was fixed. Mobilization of the malleus was performed either immediately or during a second operation.

Results

Hearing was improved dramatically in 6 ears out of 8 with an air-bone gap of less than 10 dB. This result lasts for as long as 18 years in the first operated ear (fig. 2). The other cases were followed up from 1 to 14 years postoperatively. A partial recovery of the conductive deafness was obtained in one ear after the mobilization of the malleus during a second operation; the air-bone gap was reduced from 70 to 40 dB. In another case, hearing was not improved presumably because of a malleus fixation. In

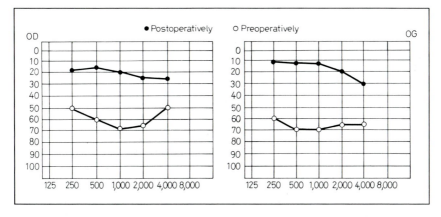

Fig. 2. Tonal audiogram of the first case operated on. The follow-up is of 18 years for the left ear and of 8 years for the right ear. Filled circles represent the postoperative and open circles the preoperative audiogram.

any case, no sensorineural hearing loss was observed. Although a slight facial paresis occurred in the first operated ear with a total recovery without sequellae, no facial falsy was then observed in the 7 other cases.

Discussion

We have operated on 4 children, boys and girls in two different families, who presented an identical, uncommon malformation of both the oval window and the facial nerve while parents in the two families were free of the disease. This congenital defect is a morphodysplasia of autosomal-recessive transmission. This occurs during the formation of the second branchial arch and the ossification of the otic capsule. The stapes are formed from the mesenchyme which grows around the stapedial artery at 4.5 weeks of embryonic development. The stapes then extends toward the otic capsule where it forms the footplate inserted into the ovalis fenestra. The Fallopian canal develops during the ninth to tenth weeks between the otic capsule and the mesenchyme, and the facial nerve runs inside the Fallopian canal. Although many malpositions of the facial nerve have been described [2, 4], the observation of the facial nerve crossing the oval window is rather uncommon and usually associated with the nondevelopment of the footplate. In most cases reported up to now, the malformation of the oval window together with the malposition of the facial nerve was unilateral so that the surgical management of this defect was not attempted. In some bilateral cases, either a fenestration of the semicircular canal [1] or a fenestration of the promontory inferior to the facial nerve [13] were performed. In all our cases which were bilateral, we have developed a surgical procedure based on our knowledge of the anatomy of the vestibule acquired during translabyrinthine approaches [12]. It is possible to drill an opening in the lateral part of the vestibule, anteriorly to the ampulla of the lateral semicircular canal without traumatizing the utricule which is at 3 mm from the lateral wall of the vestibule. Since in our observations there was, instead of the Fallopian canal, a bony area above the fossa ovalis which formed the lateral wall of the vestibule, a fenestra was drilled in this place medially to the long process of the incus and just above the malpositioned facial nerve. When the vestibulotomy was performed, a Teflon piston of either 0.4 or 0.6 mm was inserted in the vestibular fenestra and hung to the incus. This procedure has provided a long-term correction of the conductive hearing loss in 6 out of 8 ears operated on. No sensorineural hearing loss was observed, and only a transient facial palsy was noticed in the first case operated on in 1969. Partial failures of the procedure occurred because of malleus fixation.

In conclusion, the transvestibular piston in case of congenital absence of the oval window with abnormal inferior course of the facial nerve is a safe procedure which provides a good hearing result.

References

1   Fernandez, A.O.; Ronis, M.L.: Congenital absence of the oval window. A review of the literature and report of a case. Laryngoscope *74:* 186–197 (1964).
2   Gerhardt, H.J.; Otto, H.D.: The intratemporal course of the facial nerve and its influence on the development of the ossicular chain. Acta oto-lar. *91:* 567–573 (1981).
3   Gundersen, T.: Congenital malformation of the stapes footplate. Archs Otolar. *85:* 171–176 (1967).
4   Hoogland, G.A.: The facial nerve coursing across the oval window area. ORL *39:* 148–154 (1977).
5   Hough, J.V.D.: Malformations and anatomical variations seen in the middle ear during the operation for mobilization of stapes. Laryngoscope *68:* 1337–1379 (1958).
6   Hough, J.V.D.: Congenital malformation of the middle ear. Archs Otolar. *78:* 335–343 (1963).

7 Nakamura, S.; Sando, I.: Congenital absence of the oval window. Archs Otolar. *84:* 131–136 (1966).

8 Pou, J.W.: Congenital absence of the oval window. Report of two cases. Laryngoscope *73:* 384–391 (1963).

9 Pou, J.W.: Congenital anomalies of the middle ear. Laryngoscope *81:* 831–839 (1971).

10 Scheer, A.A.: Correction of congenital middle ear deformities. Archs Otolar. *85:* 269–277 (1987).

11 Sterkers, J.M.: Aplasie de la fenêtre ovale et de l'aqueduc de Fallope. Cure de la surdité par piston attico-vestibulaire. Annls Oto-Lar. *97:* 609–615 (1980).

12 Sterkers, J.M.; Desgeorges, M.; Sterkers, O.; Corlieu, P.; Viala, P.: Chirurgie du neurinome de l'acoustique et autres tumeurs du conduit auditif interne et de l'angle ponto-cérébelleux. A propos de 602 cas. Annls Oto-Lar. *103:* 487–492 (1986).

13 Tabor, J.R.: Absence of the oval window. Archs Otolar. *74:* 515–521 (1961).

Dr. Olivier Sterkers, Service d'ORL, Hôpital Beaujon,
100, boulevard du Général-Leclerc, F–92110 Clichy (France)

Secretory Otitis Media

Adv. Oto-Rhino-Laryng., vol. 40, pp. 38–46 (Karger, Basel 1988)

Definition and Character of Acute and Secretory Otitis media

Paul B. van Cauwenberge

Department of Otorhinolaryngology, State University, Ghent, Belgium

When studying and discussing the subject of otitis media, it is necessary to define the various clinical pictures belonging to middle ear inflammation, in order to avoid unnecessary contradictions and discussions. There used to be a lot of confusion with regard to the terminology of otitis media, but recently considerable effort was made to standardize the definitions and classification. Panels on 'Definition and Classification' were organized during the four International Symposia on Otitis Media with Effusion, and the results of their discussions should guide our terminology with regard to otitis media [1, 2].

It is important to note that these panels agreed to propose and define terms strictly on *clinical grounds,* excluding terms used in other disciplines such as audiology, pathology, immunology and bacteriology.

In this article we will summarize the most important aspects of definition and classification and give a survey of the results of cytological, bacteriological, immunological and biochemical examination of the effusions, illustrating in this way the character of the effusions.

Definition and Classification

One system of classification is the best guarantee to avoid misunderstanding. Of course, synonyms will always exist, as will do subclassifications. Thanks to basic research we got rid of incorrect terms such as 'sterile otitis media' and 'allergic otitis media'.

Although the Panel on Definition and Classification of the 1983 Research Conference on Recent Advances in Otitis Media with Effusion [2] stated that acceptance of terms and their definitions is voluntary, we should – in the international literature – stick to the one classification and terminology suggested by this panel, in order to facilitate communication between otologists, paediatricians and basic researchers and within these groups.

Otitis media was defined as inflammation of the middle ear. It is classified in 4 groups: (a) myringitis; (b) acute suppurative otitis media; (c) secretory otitis media (SOM); (d) chronic suppurative otitis media.

Whereas acute suppurative and chronic suppurative otitis media refer to clinically infected forms of otitis, secretory otitis media (synonym: chronic otitis media with effusion) refers to a *clinically non-infected* form of otitis media, with fluid accumulation behind an intact eardrum. In only a minority of cases of otitis media behind an intact eardrum, a distinction can be made between serous, mucoid or purulent effusions. It is, consequently, safer to use the broader terms such as acute (suppurative) otitis media or secretory otitis media before a myringotomy is performed or before a spontaneous drum perforation occurs.

Character of Effusions

Thanks to biochemical, microbiological, cytological and immunological examinations of the effusions, the true nature of the effusions can be examined and differences between the serous, mucoid and purulent forms can be detected, illustrating a different etiopathology or different stage of disease.

We will give a survey of some of these aspects.

Bacteriology

The majority (80–90%) of purulent effusions in cases of *acute otitis media* contain bacteria. The most commonly found bacterium is *Streptococcus pneumoniae* (50–60%), followed by *Haemophilus influenzae* (15–20%), *Branhamella catarrhalis* (5–15%) and *Staphylococcus epidermidis* (5–15%) [3].

For secretory otitis media the picture is somewhat different. In our own study, where 3 different staining techniques were used for direct microscopic examination, and aerobic and anaerobic culturing was per-

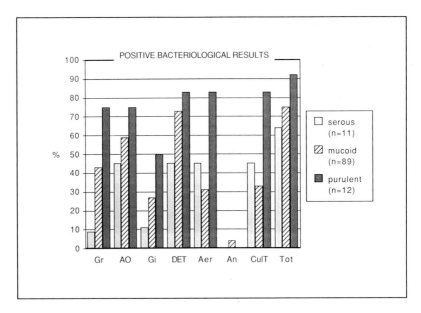

Fig. 1. Detection of bacteria by different bacteriological techniques in 112 middle ear effusions, according to the macroscopic aspect of the effusions. Gr = Gram stain; AO = acridine orange stain; Gi = Giemsa stain; DET = bacteria detected in at least one stain; Aer = aerobic culture; An = anaerobic culture; CulT = bacterial growth in at least one culture medium; Tot = detection of bacteria in smear and/or culture.

formed [4], we noted that bacteria were found in 63% of serous SOM, in 76% of mucoid SOM and in 92% of purulent SOM (fig. 1). These figures are in concordance with earlier reports [5].

When dividing the large group of mucoid effusions into 3 groups: sticky glue, normal mucus and rather liquid mucus, we noted that the glue group revealed less frequently bacteria than the normal mucus and the seromucus group, especially when culturing [4]; this sticky glue is probably the manifestation of a long lasting middle ear disease where the infectious process became less and less important and/or where anti-infectious factors (humoral and cellular) became more and more important. The identification of the bacteria by culture revealed no significant differences between the different groups of OME. *H. influenzae* was most frequently cultured (in 45% of the positive cases), followed by *S. pneumoniae* (18%), *B. catarrhalis* (16%) and micrococci (14%).

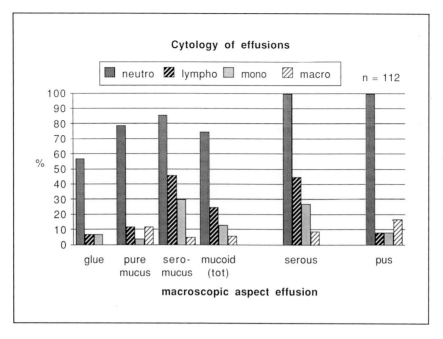

Fig. 2. Cytological findings in 112 middle ear effusions, according to the macroscopical aspect of the effusions. Neutro = Neutrophils (polymorphonucleocytes); lympho = lymphocytes; mono = monocytes; macro = macrophages.

Respiratory viral infections are important in the epidemiology of acute otitis media [6], but their role in the direct pathogenesis is less clear [7]. In a literature review [8] it was found that only 4% of middle ear effusions showed a positive culture of viruses. However, RSV antigen was detected in 19% of middle ear effusions collected at a time when RSV infection was prevalent in the community [9].

Cytology

In *acute suppurative otitis media,* polymorphonucleocytes are the predominant and nearly always the exclusive cells.

In *SOM,* the cytological findings are different in the various classes of effusions [4] (fig. 2). *Polymorphonucleocytes* are found in all purulent effusions, but also in (nearly) all serous secretions. The clear serous secretions are indeed not cell-free, because also lymphocytes and, in a lesser extent,

Table I. B and T lymphocyte populations (in %) in tonsils, blood and MEE

Monoclonal antibody	Tonsils	Blood	MEE
CD19	60 ± 16	11.6 ± 4.4	14.7 ± 12.0
CD2	37 ± 9	78.4 ± 4.3	55.8 ± 20.6
CD3	33 ± 9	68.6 ± 7.1	55.3 ± 20.5
CD4	33 ± 8	43.1 ± 5.4	32.3 ± 16.7
CD8	8 ± 4	26.7 ± 4.9	19.8 ± 12.1
CD4/CD8	4.1	1.6	1.6

CD19 = Leu 12, pan B cell marker; CD2 = OKT11, pan T, E rosette receptor; CD3 = OKT3, pan T, mature T cell; CD4 = OKT4, T helper/inducer subset; CD8 = OKT8, T suppressor/cytotoxic subset.

mononuclear cells and macrophages are found. Purulent secretions are nearly exclusively colonized by polymorphonucleocytes; the cellular picture is very similar to that of acute purulent otitis. Mucoid secretions, and especially sticky glue, reveal less frequently inflammatory cells, which may confirm that in this stage of the disease inflammatory processes are not so important anymore. Seromucous secretions give a similar cytological picture as serous secretions.

There is no uniform pattern of *lymphocytes* present in the effusions [10, 11]. Lymphocytes account for not more than 20% of the cells found in the effusions. Neutrophils are in the vast majority the predominant cells. T lymphocytes are the predominant component of the lymphocytes with a mean value of 56%. T helper/inducer lymphocytes (CD4) are in most samples more numerous (31%) than T suppressor/cytotoxic lymphocytes (CD8) (14%) [11]. The distribution of B lymphocytes and subpopulations of T lymphocytes lies in between the values for blood and tonsil/adenoid tissue, but is more similar to that of blood (table I).

There are no signs of a lack of essential cellular defense mechanisms and it is postulated that the cellular picture in mucoid OME may vary considerably depending upon the stage of the disease. There is no reason to assume that in the majority of children with mucoid otitis media the cellular immunological processes in the middle ear differ from those of chronic infections in other closed cavities of the body. *Eosinophils* and *basophils* are nearly never found in the effusions, although they are present in small quantity in the middle ear mucosa of patients with SOM.

Mucus

The largest part of the mucus is derived from the hyperplastic, secretory mucosa in which the number of goblet cells and secretory glands are numerous, whereas in a normal mucosa these elements are sparse. The mucus is not the result of transsudation or exudation, which is probably the main pathophysiological phenomenon in serous SOM.

The mucosubstances are glycoproteins containing *D*-galactose, *D*-mannose, *D*-glucose, *D*-xylose, *L*-fucose, N-acetyl-*D*-glucosamine residues, N-acetylgalactosamines and various derivates of neuraminic acid in their saccharide chains [12]. It is the presence of sugar residues that makes the secretions sticky [13].

Biochemistry

Whereas in experimental models the *total protein* concentration is about the same in the effusion as in the corresponding serum, suggesting that these effusions are pure transsudates, total protein in the middle ear effusion is higher than in serum in naturally occurring effusions in humans, suggesting that more than a pure transsudate is involved in SOM [14]. It was found that mucoid effusions contain a higher total protein than serous effusions [15].

There exists a relationship between the lipid concentration in the middle ear effusion and the duration of the disease: the longer the duration of the middle ear effusion the lower the total lipid concentration, which is only due to the decrease of the triglyceride level [15]. Total lipid was lower in mucoid effusions than in serous ones, suggesting a longer duration in this kind of effusion. The *glucose* concentration in both serous and mucoid effusions is lower than in serum, because of the increased glucose consumption by the inflammatory cells [14]. From the *electrolytes,* only potassium was found to have a higher concentration in the effusions than the serum [14]. The levels of oxidative and hydrolytic *enzymes* in middle ear effusions are generally higher than in serum, and in mucoid effusion higher than in serous secretions. In addition, the lower molecular weight enzymes (e.g. LDH and lysozyme) are relatively more abundant in middle ear effusions than the higher molecular weight enzymes such as leucine aminopeptidase and alkaline phosphatase [14]. According to the same authors the mucoid effusions reflect a higher degree of inflammatory changes. The activity of aspartate and alanine *transaminases* (GOT and GPT) is about 40 times higher in effusions than in serum [16]. This finding further corroborates the active secretory capacity of the proliferating middle ear mucosa. Mucoid effusions show a much lower *fibrinolytic activity* than serous effusions [17]. The lack of fibrinolytic activity, promoting the development of a fibrin mash, may explain the conversion of a simple middle ear effusion into mucoid SOM, and even the eventual development of adhesive otitis media. A series of *mediators of inflammation* are identified in the middle ear effusions. Among them we mention histamine, leukotactic factors, bradykinins, prostaglandins (E and F series), leukotrienes (B4 and C4), platelet activating factor (PAF), lysosomal enzymes and lysozyme [18]. In general, most mediators of inflammation appear to be significantly higher in mucoid effusions than in the serous effusion [19].

Immunoglobulins

The immunoglobulin content of the middle ear effusions demonstrates that an active secretory process with local immunoglobulin production takes place in the middle ear mucosa; there are, of course, also signs of transudation. While the IgG concentration in the middle ear effusions is similar to that of the serum, IgA and sIgA levels are much higher in the effusions than in serum. Mucoid effusions have higher levels than serous ones, suggesting a more intense active production or a more concentrated fluid [20]. Immunofluorescent studies of the middle ear mucosa demonstrated active production of IgA, IgG and IgE [21].

Although a type I hypersensitivity does not seem to play an important role in naturally occurring SOM, it is demonstrated that the IgE levels are higher in the effusions than in serum [22], but this is only true for mucoid effusions; serous effusions have a similar IgE concentration as the corresponding serum.

Conclusion

There is a variety of inflammatory processes that can take place in the middle ear cleft. This results in different clinical forms of otitis media, which all have their peculiarities in pathogenesis, symptomatology and natural history. It is obvious that active processes take place in the middle ear mucosa, and that mucoid effusions show a more intense and longer-lasting activity. The fact that the various kinds of effusions have a different prognosis, mucoid effusions giving the worst results [23], stresses the importance of identifying in each individual case the real character of the effusion.

References

1 Modified Report of the Ad Hoc Committee on Definition and Classification of Otitis Media. Ann. Otol. Rhinol. Lar. *89:* suppl. 69, pp. 6–8 (1980).

2 Definition and Classification. Ann. Otol. Rhinol. Lar. *94:* suppl. 116, pp. 8–9 (1985).

3 Lundgren, K.; Ingvarsson, L.: Microbiology of acute otitis media; in Sadé, Acute and secretory otitis media, pp. 175–179 (Kugler, Amsterdam 1986).

4 van Cauwenberge, P.; Rysselaere, M.; Waelkens, B.: Bacteriological and cytological findings according to the macroscopic characteristics of the middle ear effusions. Auris-Nasus-Larynx *12:* suppl. 1, pp. 73–76 (1985).

5 Liu, Y.S.; Lim, D.J.; Lang, R.W.; Birck, H.G.: Chronic middle ear effusions. Immunochemical and bacteriological investigations. Archs Otolar. *101:* 278–286 (1975).

6 Henderson, F.W.; Collier, A.M.; Sanyal, M.A.: A longitudinal study of respiratory viruses and bacteria in the etiology of acute otitis media with effusion. New Engl. J. Med. *306:* 1377–1380 (1982).

7 Nelson, J.D.: State of the art: microbiology of acute otitis media with effusion; in Lim, Bluestone, Klein, Nelson, Recent advances in otitis media with effusion, pp. 105–106 (Decker, Philadelphia 1985).

8 Klein, J.O.; Teele, D.W.: Isolation of viruses and mycoplasmas from middle ear effusions. A review. Ann. Otol. Rhinol. Lar. *85:* suppl. 25, pp. 140–146 (1976).

9 Klein, J.O.; Dolette, F.R.; Yolken, R.H.: The role of respiratory syncytial virus and other viral pathogens in acute otitis media. J. Pediat. *101:* 16–21 (1982).

10 Palva, T.; Taskinen, E.; Häyry, P.: T lymphocytes in secretory otitis media; in Veldman, McCabe, Huizing, Mygind, Immunobiology, autoimmunity, transplantation in otorhinolaryngology, pp. 45–50 (Kugler, Amsterdam 1985).

11 van Cauwenberge, P.; Plum, J.; de Smedt, M.: Analysis of T & B lymphocytes in middle ear effusions of children with OME; in Veldman, McCabe, Huizing, Mygind, Immunobiology in otorhinolaryngology, pp. 247–252 (Kugler, Amsterdam 1987).

12 Bernstein, J.M.; Boerst, M.; Hayes, E.R.: Mucosubstances in otitis media with effusion. Ann. Otol. Rhinol. Laryn. *88:* 334–338 (1979).

13 Meri, S.; Holthöfel, H.; Palva, T.: Characterization of mucosubstances with lectins in secretory otitis media; in Sadé, Acute and secretory otitis media, pp. 259–261 (Kugler, Amsterdam 1986).

14 Juhn, S.K.; Huff, J.S.: Biochemical characteristics of middle ear effusions. Ann. Otol. Rhinol. Lar. *85:* suppl. 25, pp. 110–116 (1976).

15 van de Calseyde, P.; Blaton, V.; Ampe, W.: The protein patterns of middle ear effusion in serous otitis media behind an intact eardrum. Acta oto-lar. *71:* 153–158 (1971).

16 Palva, T.; Nousiainen, R.; Raunio, V.: Aspartate and alanine transaminases in middle ear effusions. Acta oto-lar. *79:* 58–59 (1975).

17 Bernstein, J.M.; Steger, R.; Back, N.: The fibrinolysin system in otitis media with effusion. Am. J. Otolar. *1:* 28–33 (1979).

18 van Cauwenberge, P.; Bernstein, J.M.: Inflammatory mediators in middle ear disease, chapt. 15; in Bernstein, Ogra, Immunology of the ear, pp. 331–343 (Raven Press, New York 1987).

19 van Cauwenberge, P.: Otitis media with effusion. Functional morphology and physiopathology of the structures involved. Acta oto-rhino-lar. belg. *36:* 5–240 (1982).

20 Mogi, G.; Maeda, S.; Yoshida, T.; Watanabe, N.: Otitis media with effusion. Specific antibody activities against exotoxins in middle ear effusions. Laryngoscope *86:* 1043–1055 (1976).

21 Hussl, B.; Lim, D.J.: Experimental middle ear effusions. An immunofluorescent study. Ann. Otol. Rhinol. Lar. *83:* 332–343 (1974).

22 Lim, D.J.; Liu, Y.S.; Schram, J.; Birch, H.G.: Immunoglobulin E in chronic middle ear effusions. Ann. Otol. Rhinol. Lar. *85:* suppl. 25, pp. 117–123 (1976).

23 van Cauwenberge, P.; Cauwe, F.; Kluyskens, P.: The long-term results of the treatment with transtympanic ventilation tubes in children with chronic secretory otitis media. Int. J. pediat. Oto-rhino-lar. *1:* 109–116 (1979).

Dr. Paul van Cauwenberge, Department of Otorhinolaryngology, State University, De Pintelaan 185, B–9000 Ghent (Belgium)

Adv. Oto-Rhino-Laryng., vol. 40, pp. 47–56 (Karger, Basel 1988)

Incidence and Risk Factors of Acute Otitis media and Otitis media with Effusion in Children of Different Age Groups

G. Pestalozza, M. Romagnoli, E. Tessitore

Divisione di Otorinolaringoiatria, Ospedale dei Bambini 'V. Buzzi', Milano, Italia

Our investigation refers to the incidence and risk factors of otitis media in children submitted to ENT evaluation (halogen light otoscope, audiometry and/or tympanometry) in different countries, as they are reported by different authors.

Neonatal Age (0–30 Days)

Our personal investigations [4, 26–28] refer to a population of 300 unselected newborns from 300 consecutive births and 970 newborns (aged 1–25 days) from the Neonatal Intensive Care Unit (NICU). The incidence of otitis media (acute otitis media, AOM) in normal unselected newborns is relatively high in respect to clinical findings (3.33%). In most cases, however, it is a silent and benign disease; diagnosis is made only by means of otoscopy. The incidence of otitis media in newborns coming from NICU is definitely higher (21.1%).

It manifests itself with not specific but more evident symptoms (irritability or lethargy, prolonged crying, vomiting, seizures). Associated illnesses (jaundice, dystrophy) which require rapid and specific treatment, are often present. In order to make a correct diagnosis repeated otoscopies are required. Due to the high compliance of the eardrum of the neonate

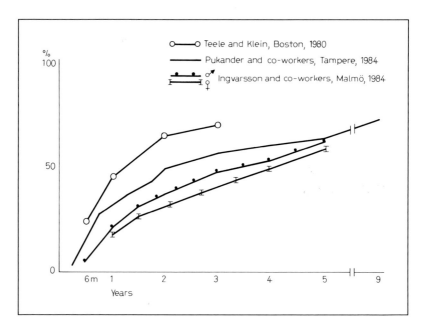

Fig. 1. Incidence of AOM in children according to age.

even in the presence of middle ear fluid, tympanometry is not a good diagnostic tool at this age. In recent studies [25, 32] it was evidenced that in the newborn when the eardrums are normal a double peak tympanogram is found. When the eardrums are congested, however, a large smooth-notched peak is more frequently found.

From 1 to 12 Months of Age

The incidence of AOM and otitis media with effusion (OME) is highest in this period of life. Symptoms are usually present, but at this age silent otitis media (AOM or OME) is still frequent. In a study on 4,582 children in Finland [29], 56,7% babies between 9 and 18 months of age suffered at least one attack of AOM (maximum prevalence at the 10th month). Similar results are referred by Ingvarsson et al. [11] on 2,404 children in Sweden (fig. 1). Marchant et al. [15] studied a group of 70 children during the first year of life. Sixty-seven percent of those children had had at least one attack of AOM.

The first episode of AOM was asymptomatic in 54% of the cases. According to a study on 2,565 children of the Boston area [12, 36], those children who have several attacks of AOM in the first months of life are more prone to recurrent purulent otitis media in infancy and consequent auditory and linguistic troubles.

From 1 to 6 Years of Age

In figure 1 it is possible to see that the incidence of attacks of AOM decreases progressively with age: at 4 years of life about 40% of children had had at least one attack of AOM. Also the incidence of OME decreases progressively and constantly with age. According to Elbrond and Birch [7] (fig. 2) type B tympanometry is 52% in the first year of life, 61% during the second year and decreases progressively to 17% at 5 years. An investigation performed in Northern Italy on 863 children [2] evidenced that after 5 years the decreased incidence of OME continues up to 12 years. Seasonal variations of the incidence of OME have been studied by several authors [3, 31, 39] and a higher incidence was demonstrated in winter (fig. 3). Results referred by Tos et al. [37, 38] also show the same trend with slightly different numbers.

From 6 to 12 Years of Age

The incidence of AOM and OME decreases constantly, as can be seen in figures 1 and 2. Incidence of serous otitis in children at 7–8 years of age is 4.2% based on otoscopy and 3% based on type B tympanometry [44]. A screening performed in Milano [16] on 18,000 school children of 7 years of age demonstrated a hearing loss > 25 dB in 4.2% of children.

Epidemiology and Risk Factors

AOM and OME are included among the most frequent diseases of childhood. It is well known that some children are more otitis prone than others: for this reason the identification of at-risk subjects is a challenge for

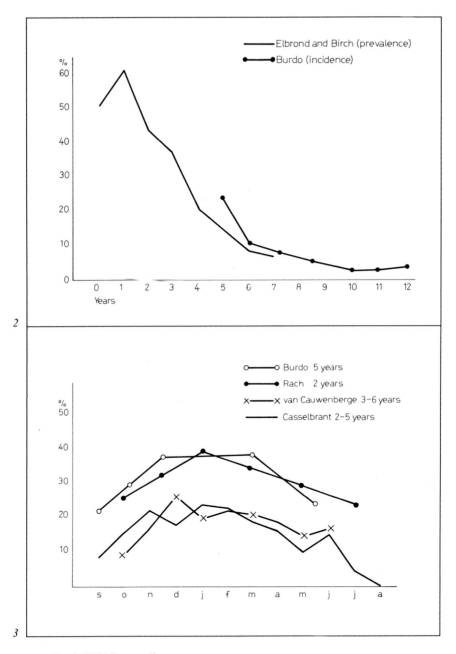

Fig. 2. TPM B according to age.
Fig. 3. Incidence of OME (TPM B) in various age groups according to season.

Table I. Identified risk factors for AOM and OME

1	Upper respiratory tract infections		
2	Winter season		
3	Hypertrophic adenoids		
4	Inadequate antibiotic treatments		
5	Genetic (including congenital malformations) and race factors		

Neonatal age	1–12 months	1–6 years	6–12 years
Meconium-stained amniotic fluid Prolonged delivery	prematurity low-birth weight early bottle feeding attending kinder-gartens and public day-care centers	attending kindergartens and preschool frequent attacks of AOM in the first year of life	the disease is less strictly related to all risk factors

	Occasional and accessory risk-factors
1	Respiratory tract infections of parents or siblings
2	Sex
3	Geographic and housing factors
4	Allergy of the study child
5	Allergy of the parents
6	Population density at home
7	Smoking of parents
8	Indoor humidification
9	Local and general immunodeficiencies

every otologist. Some predisposing factors are common to all ages, other ones are specific for some age groups. Further some risk factors are validated by personal experience and by statistical data, whereas others are not (table I).

Upper respiratory tract infections and *winter season* are obviously important. General practioners, pediatricians and otolaryngologists could not contradict this belief. In order to give a statistical basis to evidence the feelings of old clinicians, several authors investigated the incidence of otitis media in relation to these conditions in wide populations of children. According to v. Cauwenberge [40] children with only one episode of common cold per year have a 90% chance to be free of AOM in the same year; a child presenting more than 4 common colds per year, however, has only a 62% chance to be free of AOM. Edematous nasal mucous membranes with hypersecretion is strictly related to the presence of OME in 2,065 preschool children. Insofar as the role of *hypertrophic adenoids* is concerned, according to some authors [17, 34] adenoidectomy has a significant therapeutic effect on OME and recurrent AOM, whereas its absolute efficacy is not validated by others [24]. The problem of *antibiotic treatment of previous attacks of AOM* is very important. Repeated antibiotic treatments of recurrent AOM certainly reduced complications and sequelae, but we are aware that OME is greatly increased since paracentesis has been substituted by antibiotics as the first treatment of AOM. v. Cauwenberge et al. [42], however, demonstrated that there is no statistically significant difference in the incidence of OME in children who, in case of AOM, were submitted to antibiotic treatment only, antibiotic treatment + myringotomy or local treatments only. It is difficult, however, to prove the significance of these data, because nobody can state that previous antibiotic treatment was adequate or inadequate. We think this is a still open problem; antibiotic treatment, however, must be given at full dosage for not less than 7 days in any case of AOM. Insofar as *genetic and race factors* are concerned, the incidence of AOM and OME is very high in American Indians and Eskimos of Alaska (78% of cases of AOM in the second year of life) and in Australian aborigines [18, 45]. In the USA the incidence is higher in the Hispanic population [35]. In American [36], Nigerian [19] and South African [9] black children the incidence of AOM and OME is lower, probably because in the blacks there is a better function of the Eustachian tube on a genetic basis [9, 45]. In some congenital malformations such as cleft palate, OME is universal [23]. Some risk factors are specific only for some age groups.

In neonatal age (0–30 days) otitis media has always an obstetrical origin [4, 26, 27, 28]. Infection reaches the middle ear through the Eustachian tube (in the newborn it is shorter, wider and more horizontal than in the older child). AOM is more frequent in cases of prolonged delivery with early ruptured membranes (6.9% in the normal population in Italy, from 17.6% to 60% in otitis media populations) and in cases with meconium-stained amniotic fluid (14% in the normal population in Italy, from 26 to 70% in otitis media populations).

From 1 to 12 months of age specific risk is *prematurity and immaturity*; it has been demonstrated [39] that children with low birth weight

(2.3 kg) and premature infants (8–10 weeks) are twice as much at risk both for AOM and OME. Prolonged breast-feeding is considered as a protective factor against otitis media as well as against upper airways infections [5, 30], due to the more prolonged action of maternal gamma-globulins.

From 1 to 6 years of age: frequent attacks of AOM in the first year of life is considered a risk factor for recurrent purulent otitis media and OME [15, 36, 19, 39]. At present the data on this matter are not statistically significant, even though speech defects in preschool children as a consequence of early attacks of AOM are mentioned by several authors [21, 33]. In Scandinavian countries several studies [7, 8, 11, 14, 29, 30] demonstrated a higher incidence of AOM and OME in *children attending kindergartens,* public day-care centers and preschool in respect to children staying at home or in family day-care centers. These studies are significant inasmuch as they are based on repeated otoscopies and tympanometries in different periods of the year in order to avoid contamination of the results due to the seasonal variations of the disease.

Accessory and occasional risk factors do not at present have a proved statistical basis. Among those mentioned in table I we will recall the following: *Sex:* Both AOM [11] and OME [35] are supposed to be more frequent in males; no reasonable explanation, however, is given to support the data; other authors [6, 39] did not find any statistically significant difference between males and females. Insofar as *housing and geographic factors* are concerned, a higher incidence of AOM and OME is present in urban areas in respect to rural areas according to some authors [11, 29] but not according to others [43]. Probably, these differences are due to seasonal variations.

Local and/or general immunodeficiencies have been studied by many authors [1, 10, 13, 20, 22]. Clinical implications are under investigation; and they will certainly be a safe guideline for the future.

Between 6 and 12 years of age: at this age there is a progressive decrease of morbidity. Otitis media becomes increasingly independent from any risk factor, upper airways infections included. The most important risk-factor in school-age children who have attacks of AOM and prolonged periods of hearing loss due to OME, is the number of previous episodes of AOM. Mucous membrane lesions become irreversible and more sensitive to repeated bacterial infections. Epithelial metaplasia and/or invasive epidermosis may be the first stage of chronic otitis media with or without cholesteatoma.

References

1   Bernstein, G.M.; Prellner, K.; Rynnel-Dagoo, B.; Sipala, P.; Palva, T.: Otitis media: the immunological factor; in Sadé, Proc. Int. Conf. Acute and Secretory Otitis media, Jerusalem 1985, pp. 203–210 (Kugler, Amsterdam 1986).

2   Burdo, S.; Vigliani, E.; Balice, R.; Brandi, L.: Aspetti epidemiologici dell'otite media secretiva: esperienza su 2475 casi. Atti del V Congr. della Soc. It. di Otorinolar. Ped., Catania 1980 (Pozzi, Roma 1980).

3   Casselbrant, M. L.; Brostoff, L. M.; Cantekin, E. I.; Ashoff, V. M.; Bluestone, C. D.: Otitis media in children in the United States, in Sadé, Proc. Int. Conf. Acute and Secretory Otitis media, Jerusalem 1985, pp. 104–108 (Kugler, Amsterdam 1986).

4   Cioce, C.; Canubi, A.: L'otite del neonato. Ann. Lar. 76: 104–108 (1978).

5   Cunnigham, A.S.: Morbidity in breast fed and artificially fed infants, part II. J. Pediat. 95: 685–689 (1979).

6   Draper, W.L.; Secretory otitis media in children: a study on 540 children. Laryngoscope 77: 639 (1967).

7   Elbrond, O.; Birch, L.: Prospective epidemiological investigation of secretory otitis media in children attending day-care centers; in Sadé, Proc. Int. Conf. Acute and Secretory Otitis media, Jerusalem 1985, pp. 147–149 (Kugler, Amsterdam 1986).

8   Fiellau-Nikolajsen, M.: Tympanometry in 3-year-old children. Type of care as an epidemiological factor in secretory otitis media and tubal dysfunction in unselected populations of 3-year-old children. Otorhinolaryngology 4: 193–205 (1979).

9   Halama, A.R.; Voogt, G.R.; Husgrave, G.H.: Prevalence of otitis media in children in a black rural community in Venda (South Africa). Int. J. Pediat. Otorhinolar. 11: 73–77 (1986).

10 Howie, W.; Ploussard, J.; Sleyer, J.: Immunization against recurrent otitis media. Ann. Otol. Lar. 85: suppl. 25, pp. 254–258 (1976).

11 Ingvarsson, L.; Lundgren, K.; Oloffson, B.: Epidemiology of acute otitis media in children. A cohort study in an urban population; in Lim, Bluestone, Klein, Nelson, Proc. 3rd Int. Symp.: Recent advances in otitis media with effusion, Fort Lauderdale 1983, pp. 19–22 (Decker, Philadelphia 1984).

12 Klein, J.O.; Teele, D.W.; Mannos, R.; Menyuk, P.; Rosner, B.A.: Otitis media with effusion during the first three years of life and development of speech and language; in Lim, Bluestone, Klein, Nelson, Proc. 3rd Int. Symp.: Recent advances in otitis media with effusion, Fort Lauderdale 1983, pp. 332–334 (Decker, Philadelphia 1984).

13 Lim, D.J.; Liu, Y.S.; Schram, J.; Birck, H.G.: Immunoglobulin E in chronic middle ear effusion. Ann. Otol. Rhinol. Lar. 85: suppl. 25, pp. 117–123 (1979).

14 Lundgren, K.; Ingvarsson, L.; Olofsson, B.: Epidemiologic aspects in children with recurrent acute otitis media; in Lim, Bluestone, Klein, Nelson, Proc. 3rd Int. Symp.: Recent advances in otitis media with effusion, Fort Lauderdale 1983, pp. 22–25 (Decker, Philadelphia 1984).

15 Marchant, C.D.; Shurin, P.; Tutihasi, M.A.; Tuzczyk, V.A.; Wasikowski, D.E.; Feinstein, J.C.: Detection of asymptomatic otitis media in early infancy; in Lim, Bluestone, Klein, Nelson, Proc. 3rd Int. Symp.: Recent advances in otitis media with effusion, Fort Lauderdale 1983, pp. 32–33 (Decker, Philadelphia 1984).

16 Massari, F.; Mazzocca, M.; Meregalli, G.; Montabetti, E.: L'attività del Centro:

organizzazione, prevenzione, terapia, programmi futuri, in L'attività del Centro Sanitario di ortofoniatria infantile M.L. Marenzi, Milano 1986.

17 Maw, A.R.: Chronic otitis media with effusion and adenotonsillectomy: a prospective randomized controlled study; in Lim, Bluestone, Klein, Nelson, Proc. 3rd Int. Symp.: Recent advances in otitis media with effusion, Fort Lauderdale 1983, pp. 299–302 (Decker, Philadelphia 1984).

18 McCafferty, G.; et al.: A nine year study of ear disease in Australian aboriginal children. J. Lar. Otol. *99:* 119–125 (1985).

19 Miller, S.A.; Omene, J.A.; Bluestone, C.D.; Torkelson, D.W.: A point prevalence of otitis media in a Nigerian village. Int. J. Pediat. Otorhinol. *5:* 19–29 (1983).

20 Mogi, G.; Maeda, S.; Umehara, T.; et al.: Secretory IgA, serum IgA and free secretory component in middle ear effusion; in Lim, Bluestone, Klein, Nelson, Proc. 3rd Int. Symp.: Recent advances in otitis media with effusion, Fort Lauderdale 1983, pp. 147–149 (Decker, Philadelphia 1984).

21 Needlemann, H.; Menyuk: Effects of hearing loss from recurrent otitis media on speech and language development; in Jaffe, Hearing loss in children (University Park Press, Baltimore 1977).

22 Palva, T.; Reitoma, S.; Kontinnen, Y.; et al.: Inflammatory cell population in the middle ear mucosa of ears with effusion. Int. J. pediat. Otorhinolar. *3:* 71–78 (1981).

23 Paradise, J.L.; Bluestone, C.D.; Felder, H.: The universality of otitis media in 50 infants with cleft palate. Pediatrics, Springfield *44:* 35–42 (1969).

24 Paradise, J.L.; Bluestone, C.D.; Rogers, K.D.; Taylor, F.H.: Efficacy of adenoidectomy in recurrent otitis media. Historical overview and preliminary results from a randomized controlled trial. Ann. Otol. Rhinol. Lar. *89:* suppl. 68, pp. 319–321 (1980).

25 Pestalozza, G.; Cusmano, C.: Evaluation of tympanometry in diagnosis and treatment of otitis media of the newborn and of the infants. Int. J. pediat. Otorhinolar. *2:* 73–82 (1980).

26 Pestalozza, G.; Cioce, C.; Romagnoli, M.; et al.: Otitis media in newborns: long-term follow-up, cytological and bacteriological investigations, in Lim, Bluestone, Klein, Nelson, Proc. 3rd Int. Symp.: Recent advances in otitis media with effusion, Fort Lauderdale 1983, pp. 40–44 (Decker, Philadelphia 1984).

27 Pestalozza, G.; Cioce, C.; Romagnoli M.; et al.: L'otite media del neonato: studio citologico, batteriologico e risultati a distanza. Acta otorhinolar. ital. *4:* 27–47 (1984).

28 Pestalozza, G.; Cioce, C.; Romagnoli, M.; Anzalotta, S.: The incidence of otitis media in newborn infants; in Sadé, Proc. Int. Conf. Acute and Secretory Otitis media, Jerusalem 1985, pp. 139–145 (Kugler, Amsterdam 1986).

29 Pukander, J.; Sipila, M.; Karma, P.: Occurrence and risk-factors in acute otitis media; in Lim, Bluestone, Klein, Nelson, Proc. 3rd Int. Symp.: Recent advances in otitis media with effusion, Fort Lauderdale 1983, pp. 9–13 (Decker, Philadelphia 1984).

30 Pukander, J.; Sipila, M.; Kataja, M.; Karma, P.: The risk of an urban child to contract acute otitis media during the first year of life; in Sadé, Proc. Int. Conf. Acute and Secretory Otitis media, Jerusalem 1985, pp. 119, 124 (Kugler, Amsterdam 1986).

31 Rach, G.H.; Zielhuis, G.A.; Broek, P. van den: The prevalence of otitis media with effusion in two year old children in the Netherlands; in Sadé, Proc. Int. Conf. Acute and Secretory Otitis media, Jerusalem 1985, pp. 135–137 (Kugler, Amsterdam 1986).

32 Romagnoli, M.: L'otite media in età neonatale: diagnosi timpanometrica in rapporto all'otoscopia (in press).

33 Ruben, R.J.; Hansen, D.G.: Summary of discussion and recommendations made during the Workshop on otitis media and development. Ann. Otol. Rhinol. Lar. *88:* suppl. 60, pp. 107–111 (1979).

34 Sadé, J.; Fuchs, C.: Adenoids, adenoidectomy and middle ear disease. A reevaluation; in Sadé, Proc. Int. Conf. Acute and Secretory Otitis media, Jerusalem 1985, pp. 519–520 (Kugler, Amsterdam 1986).

35 Stewart, I.A.: The natural history of secretory otitis media with some observations on retraction pockets; in Sadé, Proc. Int. Conf. Acute and Secretory Otitis media, Jerusalem 1985, pp. 87–89 (Kugler, Amsterdam 1986).

36 Teele, D.W.; Klein, J.O.; Rosner, B.A.: Epidemiology of otitis media in children. Ann. Otol. Rhinol. Lar. *89:* suppl. 68, p. 5 (1980).

37 Tos, M.; Stangerup, S.-E.; Hvid, G.; Andreassen, U.K.; Thomsen, J.; Holen-Jensen, S.: Natural history of secretory otitis media; in Lim, Bluestone, Klein, Nelson, Proc. 3rd Int. Symp.: Recent advances in otitis media with effusion, Fort Lauderdale 1983, pp. 36–40 (Decker, Philadelphia 1984).

38 Tos, M.; Stangerup, S.-E.; Hvid, G.; Andreassen, U.K.; Thomsen, J.: Epidemiology and natural history of secretory otitis; in Sadé, Proc. Int. Conf. Acute and Secretory Otitis media, Jerusalem 1985, pp. 95–106 (Kugler, Amsterdam 1986).

39 v. Cauwenberge, P.B.; Kluyskens, P.M.: Some predisposing factors in otitis media with effusion; in Lim, Bluestone, Klein, Nelson, Proc. 3rd Int. Symp.: Recent advances in otitis media with effusion, Fort Lauderdale 1985, pp. 28–32 (Decker, Philadelphia 1984).

40 v. Cauwenberge, P.B.: Otitis media in relation to other upper respiratory tract infections; in Sadé, Proc. Int. Conf. Acute and Secretory Otitis media, Jerusalem 1985, pp. 129–139 (Kugler, Amsterdam 1986).

41 v. Cauwenberge, P.B.: Relevant and irrelevant predisposing factors in secretory otitis media. Acta oto-lar., suppl. 4141, pp. 147–153 (1984).

42 v. Cauwenberge, P.B.; Declerq, G.; Kluyskens, P.M.: The relationship between acute and secretory otitis media; in Sadé, Proc. Int. Conf. Acute and Secretory Otitis media, Jerusalem 1985, pp. 77–82 (Kugler, Amsterdam 1986).

43 v. Cauwenberge, P.B.: The character of acute and secretory otitis media; in Sadé, Proc. Int. Conf. Acute and Secretory Otitis media, Jerusalem 1985, pp. 1–11 (Kugler, Amsterdam 1986).

44 Virolainen; et al.: Prevalence of secretory otitis media in seven to eight year old school children Ann. Otol. Rhinol. Lar. *89:* suppl. 68, pp. 7–10 (1980).

45 Wiet, R.J.; De Blanc, G.B.; Stewart, J.; Weider, D.J.: Natural history of otitis media in the American native. Ann. Otol. Rhinol. Lar. *89:* suppl. 68, pp. 14–19 (1980).

G. Pestalozza, MD, Divisione di Otorinolaringoiatria,
Ospedale dei Bambini 'V. Buzzi', Via Castelvetro 32, I-20100 Milano (Italy)

Adv. Oto-Rhino-Laryng., vol. 40, pp. 57–64 (Karger, Basel 1988)

Etiologic Factors in Secretory Otitis

M. Tos

ENT Department, Gentofte University Hospital, Hellerup, Denmark

Clinically, the etiology of secretory otitis is a complex and multifarious issue. Infection, tubal dysfunction and allergy are conditions often pointed out as the most important etiologic factors, which may replace or reinforce each other [1–12]. As the exact time of occurrence of secretory otitis cannot be determined in children, retrospective clinical studies are not well suited to disclose what is the cause and what is the effect of the disease.

We have performed repetitive tympanometry prospectively in three cohorts of otherwise healthy children and have currently analyzed the etiology factors contributing to deterioration and improvement of the tympanometric conditions.

Patients and Method

Cohort I comprises 150 children born consecutively from January to April 1977 in the maternity ward of the Gentofte Hospital. Tympanometry was first performed immediately after birth [1, 2] and repeated every 3 months until the age of 2 years, and then annually until the age of 8 years. In all, tympanometry was performed 15 times [3].

Cohort II comprises 278 healthy children born during the first 10 days of every month in 1976 in two municipalities of the Copenhagen county with 120,000 inhabitants. Tympanometry was first performed at the age of 2 years in November 1977 [4], and then repeated every third month until August 1978 [5–7], and again 6 months later in February 1979; from then on tympanometry was performed annually until the age of 9 years. In all, 11 examinations have been performed.

Cohort III originally comprised 373 healthy 4-year-old children born during the first 10 days of every month in 1975 in two other municipalities of the Copenhagen County with a total of 130,000 inhabitants [13, 14] Tympanometry was first performed at the age of 4 years in February 1979, and repeated every third month until February 1980 and since then annually until the age of 10; in all, tympanometry was performed 10 times in this group [3].

Each examination included otoscopy and tympanometry, and the past history as well as otologic diseases between trials were carefully recorded.

Table I. Incidence of URI during the preceding 3-month periods related to tympanometry at 6, 9 and 12 months of age

Tympanogram type/age	% of ears			
	none	few	many	total
Types at 6 months	URI during 3–6 months of age			
	(n = 172)	(n = 108)	(n = 46)	(n = 326)
A	72	59	48	61
C_1	22	32	28	28
C_2	6	8	17	9
B	–*	1	7	2
Types at 9 months	URI during 6–9 months of age			
	(n = 8)	(n = 94)	(n = 134)	(n = 236)
A	100	63	35	48
C_1	–	25	48	37
C_2	–	12***	10	11
B	–	1	7	4
Types at 12 months	URI during 9–12 months of age			
	(n = 8)	(n = 68)	(n = 102)	(n = 178)
A	75	50	31	40
C_1	25	28	28	28
C_2	–	19***	22	20
B	–	3	19	12

* $p < 0.05$; *** $p < 0.001$.
*** Between first and third columns.

Upper Respiratory Tract Infections (URI)

URI in Infancy

At birth tympanometry was completely normal [1]. From birth to the age of 1 year, a considerable deterioration of the tubal function took place; thus, 13% had type B tympanograms at 12 months [2]. The principal causes of deterioration were catarrhalia and URI, the incidence of which gradually increased during infancy.

During the first 3 months of life, 23% of the children in cohort I had URI, and tympanometry at 3 months showed type A in 70%, C_1 in 28% and C_2 in 2%. These values are significantly poorer (χ^2 test, p < 0.002) than those obtained among children who had not had URI during that period (type A in 80% and C_1 in 14%).

During the ensuing 3 months (table I), the number of children having URI increased, and the distribution of tympanogram types showed poorer conditions in these children than in those who had not had URI during the preceding period. The difference is especially marked between children having had a few episodes of URI and those having had many episodes (table I).

URI at Age 2–3

For the 2-year-old children in cohort II the best tympanograms were at all trials found among those who had not had URI during the preceding 3 months. The tympanometric conditions were significantly poorer in children having had few episodes of URI and poorest in those with many episodes of URI (table II).

As has been shown previously [3–7], the tympanogram type changed from one trial to another and could to a high degree be correlated to the change in incidence of URI during the period preceding the trial (table III). Thus, the best tympanograms were found among children with a declining incidence of URI and among those who had not had URI for a considerable period. The poorest tympanograms occurred among those with an increasing incidence of URI and among children who had had many episodes of URI during the preceding 6 months.

The distribution of tympanograms is greatly influenced by the presence and severity of URI at the time of screening. Among the 2-year-old children who at the trial in February 1978 [5] had severe URI, 41% had type B tympanograms compared with 7% among those who did not suffer from URI at the time of examination.

Table II. Relationship between incidence of URI in two year-old children and tympanogram types

Tympanogram types	Incidence of URI, % of ears			
	none	few	many	total
November 1977	Autumn 1977			
	(n = 64)	(n = 402)	(n = 90)	(n = 556)
A	78	50	27	50
C_1	14	21	16	19
C_2	3	19	36	20
B	5***	9***	22	11
May 1978	Spring 1978			
	(n = 130)	(n = 236)	(n = 114)	(n = 480)
A	87	48	21	52
C_1	11	31	16	22
C_2	2	14	31	15
B	1***	7***	32	11

*** $p < 0.001$.

URI at Age 4–6

In cohort III [13, 14] an increased incidence of URI resulted in deterioration of the tympanogram types; thus, in 60% of ears the type deteriorated to either C_2 or B. Conversely, children with a declining incidence of URI showed an improvement to type C_1 or A in 66% of the ears [14]. The tympanometric conditions were significantly poorest in children suffering from URI at the time of study [14].

URI and Internal Tubal Occlusion

In URI, catarrhalia, and acute rhinopharyngitis, several pathoanatomical manifestations are present each of which may exert an influence on the middle ear ventilation and the middle ear pressure.

Table III. Alteration of tympanogram types in 2-year-old children between two screenings related to change in frequency of URI in the periods before the screenings

Changes of tympanograms	Frequency of URI, % of ears				
	increased	decreased	unchanged		
			none	few	many
	November 1977–February 1978				
	(n = 78)	(n = 118)	(n = 30)	(n = 230)	(n = 52)
Unchanged A or C_1	30	70	97	56	24
Improved to A or C	5	23		14	12
Deteriorated to C_2 or B	33***	2	3	14***	17
Unchanged, C_2 or B	32	5		17	48
	February 1978–May 1978				
	(n = 126)	(n = 134)	(n = 36)	(n = 140)	(n = 44)
Unchanged A or C_1	51	64	92	56	23
Improved to A or C_1	7	26	8	21	21
Deteriorated to C_2 or B	16**	2		11***	2
Unchanged C_2 or B	26	8		12	55

** $p < 0.01$; *** $p < 0.001$.

(1) Nasal stenosis and reduced ventilation of the rhinopharynx give rise to a negative middle ear pressure, as we have demonstrated in patients subjected to nasotracheal intubation [15].

(2) A reduced air-flow through the rhinopharynx causes accumulation of mucus, which may promote infection of the tubal mucosa.

(3) In URI, edema of the mucosa may spread to the tubal mucosa resulting in internal tubal occlusion. Involvement of the tubal mucosa causes stasis of the mucociliary flow and promotes an ascending bacterial infection of the middle ear mucosa. In temporal bones from children with secretory otitis, we have found distinct inflammatory changes of the mucosa of the Eustachian tube [16]. The constant alteration of the venti-

lation of the middle ear, which in all available studies of children of different ages has been shown to be correlated to URI, results from changes in tubal patency which in turn are determined by inflammatory processes brought about by reversible changes of the tubal mucosa and changes of the air-flow in the rhinopharynx [15–17].

(4) During an episode of URI, swelling of the lymphoid tissue in the rhinopharynx impairs the ventilation of the middle ear, either directly in the form of external tubal occlusion, or indirectly as blockage of the air-flow in the rhinopharynx. In mononucleosis infectiosa [17], we demonstrated a negative middle ear pressure in 90% of the patients during the first week. The pressure gradually normalized in step with recovery of nasal stenosis and abatement of lymphoid tissues swelling in the rhinopharynx [17].

Acute Suppurative Otitis

Of the 2-year-old children having had acute suppurative otitis before the first trial, 18% had a type B tympanogram compared with 9% among children with no prior history of otitis. However, children with previous attacks of acute otitis had also had URI [7]. A similar, significant correlation between acute suppurative otitis and secretory otitis was also demonstrated among the 4-year-old children of cohort III [18].

Analysis of the tympanogram types before and after acute otitis showed [19] that this disease has an impairing effect on the tubal function. It is, however, not the most dominating etiologic factor in as much as secretory otitis occurs in a high percentage of ears never having had acute otitis (11%). The close correlation between acute otitis and secretory otitis is attributable to the fact that acute otitis is just as often the result of secretory otitis as it is the cause of it [19].

Other Etiologic Factors

Bacteria in the Rhinopharynx

Among the 2-year-old healthy children of cohort II, a pathologic flora was found in 32% [7]. The tympanometric conditions were significantly poorer in this group than among children having a normal flora. The most common bacteria were *Haemophilus influenzae* (13%), pneumococci (9%), and *Staphylococcus aureus* (5%).

In another analysis of the rhinopharyngeal flora in children aged 4–6 years from all three cohorts [20], a normal flora was found in a significantly higher percentage of healthy children (type A or C_1 at three trials) compared with those suffering from secretory otitis (type B or C_2 at three consecutive trials).

Streptococcus pneumoniae was significantly more frequent in children with secretory otitis (49%) than in healthy children (23%), indicating that this bacteria plays an important role in the etiology of secretory otitis [20].

Adenoid Vegetations

In cohort III, inspection of the rhinopharynx revealed enlarged adenoid vegetations in 93 (25%) of the children aged 4 years. The tympanometric conditions in these children were significantly poorer ($p < 0.001$) (type B in 22%) than in 280 children with no enlargement of the adenoid vegetations (type B in 10%) [18].

Allergy

No positive correlation could be established between allergy and secretory otitis [18]. This applied both to the 2-year-old children in cohort II [7], of whom 30 showed clinical signs of allergy, and to the 4-year-old children of cohort III, of whom 51 had a history of allergy.

Predisposition

A type B tympanogram occurred in 10% of children with a predisposition to otitis media from both parents; in 7% of children with predisposition from one parent only, and in 12% of children with no predisposition [7].

Children's Diseases

Measles, rubeola, whooping cough, and varicella did not influence the distribution of tympanogram types or the incidence of secretory otitis and neither did tonsillitis or subglottic laryngitis [7, 18].

References

1   Poulsen, G.; Tos, M.: Screening tympanometry in newborn infants and during the first six months of life. Scand. Audiol. *7:* 159–166 (1978).

2   Tos, M.; Poulsen, G.; Hancke, A.B.: Screening tympanometry during the first year of life. Acta oto-lar. *88:* 388–394 (1979).

3   Tos, M.; Stangerup, S.-E.; Hvid, G.; Andreassen, U.K.; Thomsen, J.: Epidemiology

of natural history of secretory otitis, in Sadé, Acute and secretory otitis media, pp. 95–106 (Kugler, Amsterdam 1986).

4 Tos, M.; Poulsen, G.; Borch, J.: Tympanometry in two-year-old children. ORL *40:* 77–85 (1978).

5 Tos, M.; Poulsen, G.; Borch, J.: Tympanometry in two-year-old children. Changes of tympanograms at the reevaluation. ORL *40:* 206–215 (1978).

6 Poulsen, G.; Tos, M.: Repetitive tympanometric screenings of two-year-old children. Scand. Audiol. *9:* 21–28 (1980).

7 Tos, M.; Poulsen, G.; Borch, J.: Etiological factors in secretory otitis. Archs Otolar. *105:* 582–588 (1979).

8 Cauwenberge, P.B. v.: Otitis media in relation to other upper respiratory tract infections; in Sadé, Acute and secretory otitis media, pp. 129–134 (Kugler, Amsterdam 1986).

9 Cauwenberge, P.B. v.; Declerco, G.; Kluyskens, P.M.: The relationship between acute and secretory otitis media; in Sadé, Acute and secretory otitis media, pp. 77–82 (Kugler, Amsterdam 1986).

10 Stewart, I.; Kirkland, C.; Simpson, A.; Silva, P.; Williams, S.: Some factors of possible etiologic significance related to otitis media with effusion; in Lim, Bluestone, Klein, Nelson, Recent advances in otitis media with effusion (Decker, Philadelphia 1984).

11 Kaneko, Y.; Okitsu, T.; Sakuma, M.; Shibahara, Y.; Yuasa, R.; Takasaka, T.; Kawamoto, K.: Incidence of secretory otitis media after acute inflammation of the middle ear cleft and the upper respiratory tract; in Lim, Bluestone, Klein, Nelson, Recent advances in otitis media with effusion (Decker, Philadelphia 1984).

12 Grote, J.J.; Kuypers, W.: Middle ear effusion and sinusitis. J. Lar. Otol. *94:* 177 (1980).

13 Tos, M.; Holm-Jensen, S.; Sørensen, C.H.; Mogensen, C.: Spontaneous course and frequency of secretory otitis in four-year-old children. Archs Otolar. *108:* 4–10 (1982).

14 Plate, S.; Sørensen, C.H.; Holm-Jensen, S.; Tos, M.: Catarrhalia as a risk factor in the development of secretory otitis media in preschool children. Acta oto-lar., suppl. 386, pp. 137–138 (1982).

15 Tos, M.; Bonding, P.: Middle-ear pressure during and after prolonged nasotracheal and nasogastric intubation. Acta oto-lar. *83:* 353–359 (1977).

16 Tos, M.: Pathology of the Eustachian tube. Ann. Otol. Rhinol. Lar. *94:* suppl. 120, pp. 17–18 (1985).

17 Bonding, P.; Tos, M.: Middle ear pressure during pathological conditions of short duration of the nose and throat. Acta oto-lar. *92:* 63–69 (1981).

18 Sørensen, C.H.; Holm-Jensen, S.; Tos, M.: Middle-ear effusion and risk factors. J. Otolar. *11:* 46–51 (1982).

19 Stangerup, S.-E.; Tos, M.: Etiological role of acute suppurative otitis media in chronic secretory otitis. Am. J. Otol. *6:* 126–131 (1985).

20 Sørensen, C.H.; Andersen, L.P.; Tos, M.; Thomsen, J.; Holm-Jensen, S.: Nasopharyngeal bacteriology and secretory otitis media. A prevalence study. Acta oto-lar. (in press, 1987).

M. Tos, MD, ENT Department, Gentofte University Hospital,
DK–2900 Hellerup (Denmark)

Adv. Oto-Rhino-Laryng., vol. 40, pp. 65–69 (Karger, Basel 1988)

Predisposing Factors for Otitis media with Effusion in Young Children

G.A. Zielhuis[a], *G.H. Rach*[b], *P. van den Broek*[b]

Departments of [a]Epidemiology and [b]Otorhinolaryngology,
University of Nijmegen, The Netherlands

Introduction

Risk factors are studied for several reasons. It might give clues for better understanding of the etiology of the disease which may direct to possibilities for primary prevention. Secondly, in case a screening is considered for the disease, knowledge of risk factors may give rise to the definition of high-risk groups that should get priority in such a screening program.

There is a large body of literature on the topic of risk indicators for OME. The variety of hypothesized risk factors include upper respiratory tract infections, childhood diseases, demographic factors, environmental factors, medical care and life style. Some of these are reasonably well documented by properly designed studies. Others are not.

We had the opportunity to study several of these factors in a large-scale epidemiologic study on the natural history of otitis media with effusion (OME) in preschool children in the city of Nijmegen.

Population and Methods

The Nijmegen project started in 1984 with a screening of a complete cohort of 2-year-old children living in the city of Nijmegen. This meant a total group of 1,439 children of this age. With 3-monthly intervals tympanometry was performed until the children became 4 years of age. All measurements were done by trained assistants at the children's home address. In the nine consecutive sessions the parents were also asked about relevant events in the period before measurements. These include potential risk factors for OME.

For reasons of clarity the risk factor analysis is limited to the fifth screening round, that is when the children were exactly 3 years of age. For the same reason all factors are rearranged to simple dichotomized variables: exposed versus not exposed, and those who have a type B tympanogram according to Jerger's classification in one or both ears and those who have not.

The relative risk (or risk ration) is used as a measure of relation.

Results

The results of the univariate analysis are shown in table I. It can be seen that gender is not a risk factor in this data set, nor are the variables related to birth and family history. Non-caucasian children seem to be of a higher risk as well as those who have older siblings.

As is expected, upper respiratory tract infections enhance the risk for OME. Particularly simple common cold and coughing at time of measurement or in the near past make a major contribution to the risk for OME. Acute and chronic otitis media ('running ear') do also enhance the risk. The same is true for symptoms of adenoiditis, such as open mouth breathing, snoring and bad breath.

Hearing loss at infants age also seems to be of some prognostic value for otitis media at the age of 3. This regards the impression of hearing loss by the parents, as well as the result of the first Ewing screening test at the age of 9 months. Finally, the use of antibiotics, bottle feeding and passive smoking are not related to OME. Children who attend public nurseries (in most cases twice a week) have a slightly higher risk for the disease.

All associations appear in the risk ratio range of 1 to 2. Of the 30 variables studied 18 showed a significant deviation from unity. Because of intercorrelations between these variables multivariate logistic regression analysis is performed to get a clear picture of the risk contribution for each of these factors themselves. The dependent variable in this case is the risk of OME.

Table II shows the results of the full analysis, that is when all 18 risk factors are entered in the model. Because of the large number of missing values for the results of the Ewing screening test this factor is not taken in the analysis. Only six factors give an independent significant contribution to the prediction of the probability of OME at the age of 3. When these six main predictors are taken in a new logistic model (table III) similar regression coefficients are found. The accompanying risk ratios, which are now adjusted for the contribution of the other five factors, are in the range of 1.5 to 2.

Although a recent history of acute otitis media is entered in the model in second instance, it appears to be the strongest independent risk factor with a risk ratio of 2.2.

Table I. Risk factors for OME (univariate; yes/no (y/n) if not otherwise stated)

Risk factor	n	% at risk	RR	95% CI
Gender (M/F)	1,050	50	0.99	0.82–1.19
Race (non-caucasian/caucasian)	1,136	9	1.29	1.05–1.59
Birthweight ($< 2,500$ g/$\geq 2,500$ g)	1,046	9	1.22	0.92–1.61
Premature birth (≥ 3 weeks y/n)	997	7	1.24	0.90–1.71
Family size (siblings y/n)	1,137	68	1.46	1.23–1.74
Birth order (older sibling y/n)	1,137	54	1.53	1.32–1.78
Acute OME in family (y/n)	890	69	1.09	0.92–1.30
OME in family (y/n)	764	49	1.15	0.97–1.35
Chronic otitis media in family (y/n)	790	15	0.79	0.61–1.02
Acute otitis media (y/n)	1,044	18	1.96	1.63–2.35
Chronic otitis media (y/n)	1,049	4	1.72	1.24–2.37
Throat infections (y/n)	1,032	13	1.10	0.84–1.44
Influenza (y/n)	1,039	20	1.18	0.95–1.46
Lower respiratory infections (y/n)	1,050	4	1.09	0.78–1.19
Severe common cold (y/n)	1,049	67	1.91	1.50–2.43
Common cold at time of measurement (y/n)	1,050	39	2.05	1.71–2.47
Coughing (y/n)	1,048	50	1.46	1.21–1.76
Coughing at time of measurement (y/n)	1,050	25	1.90	1.59–2.27
Open mouth at day-time (y/n)	1,068	11	1.76	1.44–2.15
Open mouth at night (y/n)	1,013	15	1.38	1.12–1.70
Snoring (y/n)	1,065	11	1.64	1.33–2.02
Restless sleep (y/n)	1,085	18	1.37	1.13–1.65
Slobbering (y/n)	1,083	8	1.30	1.00–1.69
Bad breath (y/n)	1,075	3	1.67	1.18–2.37
Hearing loss at infants age (y/n)	1,105	3	1.75	1.37–2.23
Ewing test (positive/negative)	912	8	1.68	1.37–2.07
History of antibiotics (y/n)	1,050	11	0.82	0.59–1.15
Breastfeeding (n/y)	1,129	30	1.03	0.89–1.21
Passive smoking (y/n)	1,093	65	1.07	0.90–1.26
Public nursery (y/n)	1,050	67	1.26	1.03–1.56

Table II. Risk factors for OME (logistic regression; dependent variable: uni- or bilateral OME)

Risk factor	Regression coefficient	p-value
Intercept	−1.88	0.04
Race	0.11	0.73
Family size	0.40	0.11
Birth order	−0.36	0.14
OME in family	0.67	0.00
Acute otitis media	0.93	0.00
Chronic ototis media	0.18	0.65
Common cold	0.44	0.04
Common cold at time of measurement	0.55	0.00
Coughing	−0.06	0.75
Coughing at time of measurement	0.82	0.00
Mouth breathing, daytime	0.53	0.06
Mouth breathing, night	0.20	0.45
Snoring	0.24	0.39
Restless sleep	−0.08	0.72
Slobbering	−0.31	0.38
Bad breath	0.27	0.55
Hearing loss before 2 years	−0.50	0.31
Public nursery	0.26	0.18

$n = 824$; $r^2 = 0.088$.

Table III. Logistic regression; risk ratio for six risk factors conditionally on the others (reference = negative on all factors)

	Beta	RR	95% CI
Common cold at time of measurement	0.67	1.73	1.31–2.29
Acute otitis media	1.02	2.23	1.68–2.95
OME in family	0.65	1.71	1.33–2.20
Coughing at time of measurement	0.66	1.71	1.27–2.30
Mouth breathing daytime	0.59	1.63	1.14–2.44
Common cold in history	0.43	1.43	1.07–1.90

$n = 980$; $r^2 = 0.102$.

Discussion

It should be emphasized that all risk factors in this study are measured by questionnaires, that is, the reliability of the answers depends on the memory of the parents of these 3-year-old children. This may have caused some measurement error which by definition reduces the risk ratios. On the other hand, this analysis gives a fairly complete picture of the total risk factor set that is suggested by the literature.

We might conclude that the contribution of these factors to the prediction of OME is low. Even the complete set of 18 risk factors (showing a significant effect in univariate analysis) only account for less than 10% of the variance in the probability of disease. This reduces the possibility for effective primary prevention by manipulation of one or more of these factors. Also, the idea of limiting an eventual screening program to some high-risk group can be put aside.

And lastly the efficacy of taking a complete medical and social history in the process of diagnosing OME in preschool children can be questioned. If so doing, the questions may better be limited to questions about earaches, common cold, habitual mouth breath and middle ear diseases in the family.

G.A. Zielhuis, PhD, Department of Epidemiology, University of Nijmegen, NL–6500 HB Nijmegen (The Netherlands)

Adv. Oto-Rhino-Laryng., vol. 40, pp. 70–80 (Karger, Basel 1988)

Complications of Acute Otitis media in Children

C.R. Pfaltz

Department of ORL, University Hospital of Basel, Basel, Switzerland

Introduction

Otogenic complications have become infrequent because antibiotic therapy has altered the course of otitis media. This statement may be found in many modern textbooks on otology. Does it really correspond with the facts of the actual situation?

Paparella et al. [1986] report that despite great advances in chemotherapy and preventive health care an increased incidence of *Haemophilus influenzae* meningitis has been demonstrated over the last few decades in many areas of the USA, Canada, England and Denmark. The increase in incidence of up to 3–400% was described by many reporters as unexplained. In a previous paper [Pfaltz and Griesemer, 1984] we were able to show that otogenic complications still occur, that they represent even today a severe medical problem and that the severity of its symptoms is often underrated or misinterpreted by the inexperienced physician.

The incidence figures for acute otitis media in Swedish children under 15 years of age amount to 10,000 per annum; the average number of acute mastoiditis of 2 per annum, resulting in a 0.02% overall incidence of complications [Prellner and Rydell, 1985]. Palva et al. [1985] reported a mastoiditis incidence of 0.04% with reference to acute otitis media. The complication rate in case of an acute mastoiditis, however, varies between 8 and 12% [Pfaltz and Griesemer, 1984; Ginsburg et al., 1980]. Hence, it may be concluded that otogenic complications, caused by oto-mastoiditis, still represent an important clinical problem, particularly in children.

Acute otitis media indicates an active inflammation due to an infection of the middle ear space of recent onset or resurgence [Scheydt and Kavanagh, 1986]. It is not a static condition but develops over a relatively short distance of time, and either resolves spontaneously or with treatment, or progresses to various other pathologic conditions. The most common complication of an acute otitis media is extension of the disease into the mastoid antrum and air cells, termed as *mastoiditis* or *oto-mastoiditis*. Definition and pathology of mastoiditis is a long-standing problem in otology. An acute infection and inflammation of the middle ear cleft involves from the very beginning an acute exsudative inflammation of the air-cell system of the temporal bone, which is not yet associated with bone resorption, i.e. osteolysis of the mastoid bone itself. This first stage may be termed *'mucosal or concomitant mastoiditis'*. As a rule rapid recovery follows adequate treatment of the primary acute otitis media.

In case of a severe and virulent infection the exsudative inflammation becomes purulent. Ulceration and necrosis of the mucosal layer occurs and if the inflammatory process is prolonged the formation of a polypoid mucosa and of granulation tissue is observed. We may term this stage *'granulomatous-exudative mastoiditis'*. This form turns into the final stage of *osteolytic mastoiditis* or *osteitis mastoidea*. It is characterized by demineralization of the bone and osteoclastic activity, causing cell partition necrosis and presenting a *'rarefying osteitis'* of the mastoid [Schuknecht, 1974]. It corresponds more or less with the clinical term of *'coalescent mastoiditis'*, describing the pathologic process as seen grossly at surgery (disappearance of previously normal cell boundaries) [Goodhill, 1979].

Otogenic complications due to mastoiditis, may develop by extension of the infection: (1) by continuity (per continuitatem); (2) by spreading along preformed routes into the intracranial space or into the lateral sinus; (3) by invasion of the labyrinth.

According to an extensive survey on 335 cases of mastoiditis [Samuel et al., 1986] the most common intracranial complications are: meningitis (38%) and in this group 80.7% under the age of 15 years, with a mortality rate of 8%; brain abscess (23.6%), 75% younger than 15 years, mortality rate 36%; extradural empyema (22%) 80% younger than 15 years, mortality rate 4%; lateral sinus thrombosis (17.4%) 82% younger than 15 years, mortality rate 10%.

This report is based on a 5-year observation period (1978–1983) made at King Edward VIII Hospital in Durban, South Africa. It refers to a population of African blacks, where otitis media is neglected and patients are reluctant to seek medical attention. This survey is therefore a reminder of the problem which is prevalent in many parts of the world in lower socio-economic groups.

Table I. Complications of mastoiditis

	Children (n = 10/98 = 10%)		Adults (n = 24/65 = 37%)	
	n	%	n	%
Meningitis	4	4	6	9
Labyrinthine fistula	3	3	4	6
Facial palsy	2	2	8	12
Sinus thrombosis	1	1	0	
Labyrinthitis	0		6	9

In the present study we should like to compare the nature and the incidence of otogenic complications in a group of 98 children (51 infants – 47 between 1 and 12 years) with those observed at our department during the same period (1979–1986) in a group of 65 adults.

Results

The *incidence of complications* is higher in adults (37%; table I) than in children (10%; table I). The difference is statistically significant (p > 0.02 < 0.05). Labyrinthitis does not occur in children and sinus thrombosis was not observed in adults. Facial palsy is a more frequent complication in adults (12%) than in children (2%).

Bacteriological Findings. On the whole the ratio between positive and negative cases does not differ significantly in the 2 age groups (table II). In children results are positive in 33%, in adults in 51% (difference statistically nonsignificant, i.e. p < 0.2 > 0.1). The isolates of the positive test cultures did not show marked discrepancies with respect to their incidence but always a mixed flora (table III). *Haemophilus influenzae,* however, was found only in children (1 infant of less than 1 year and 1 child of 2 years).

Otoscopic Findings and Histological Diagnosis (table IV). Spontaneous perforations occur more frequently in adults (34%) than in children (10%);

Table II. Bacteriological findings in children (n = 70) and adults (n = 49)

Type of mastoiditis	Children				Adults			
	positive		negative		positive		negative	
	n	%	n	%	n	%	n	%
Acute	13	19	14	20	10	20	8	16
Subacute	10	14	33	47	15	31	16	33

Table III. Bacteriology

	Acute mastoiditis	Subacute mastoiditis
Adults	Pneumococci Enterobacter *Staphylococcus albus* Pseudomonas	*Staphylococcus aureus* Pneumococci Proteus Pseudomonas
Children	Pneumococci *S. albus*	*S. aureus* Pseudomonas

Table IV. Correlation: otoscopic findings/histological diagnosis

Otoscopic finding (tympanic membrane)	Granulomatous mastoiditis		Osteolytic mastoiditis		Concomitant mastoiditis	
	n	%	n	%	n	%
Children (n = 98)						
Normal	5	5	5	5	5	5
Hyperemic	13	13	13	13	7	8
Blurred landmarks	11	11	13	13	0	
Spontaneous perforation	10	10	11	12	5	5
Adults (n = 59)						
Normal	1	2	1	2	1	2
Hyperemic	5	8	5	8	3	5
Blurred landmarks	8	14	3	5	0	
Spontaneous perforation	20	34	9	15	3	5

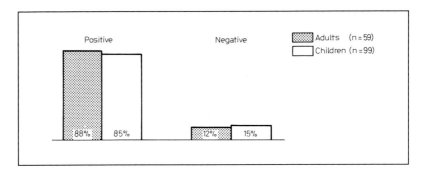

Fig. 1. Radiological findings in mastoiditis.

the other pathologic otoscopic findings do not demonstrate any significant difference between the 2 age groups.

Radiological Findings (fig. 1; table V). In both groups pathological X-rays of the temporal bone could be demonstrated in the majority of the cases (88% in adults, 85% in children). There was no difference between the 2 age groups with respect to the severity of the otoscopic symptoms in relation with the diagnostic importance of the radiological signs.

Correlation between Severity of Radiological Symptoms and Histological Findings (table VI). Radiologically, false positives were extremely rare in both age groups (1–2%) and equally false negatives (approximately 5% for both groups). The most striking difference between the two age groups could be found with respect to the *interval between the onset of the otitis media and the clinical manifestation of the oto-mastoiditis* (fig. 2).

In the group of children the incidence of mastoiditis (fig. 2) reaches a peak between the third and the sixth month after the onset of the otitis media whereas in the group of adults more complications (mastoiditis) are observed between the first and the fourth week (difference between the 2 groups statistically significant: p < 0.01 > 0.001). Another difference between the two age groups concerns the *manifestation of unspecific symptoms* indicating the presence of an inflammatory focus (table VII). These unspecific symptoms which are prevalent in infants were the first important signs leading to the final diagnosis in 60% of all the cases within the children's group. Mortality of complications was *nil* in both groups.

Table V. Correlation: X-ray/otoscopic findings

Otoscopic finding	X-ray negative		X-ray positive	
	n	%	n	%
Children (n = 98)				
Normal	4	4	11	11
Hyperemic tympanic membrane	3	3	30	30
Blurred tympanic landmarks	2	2	23	23
Spontaneous perforation	5	6	21	21
Total	14	15	84	85
Adults (n = 59)				
Normal	1	2	3	5
Hyperemia	2	3	11	19
Blurred landmarks	3	5	8	13
Spontaneous perforation	1	2	30	51
Total	7	12	52	88

Table VI. Correlation: X-ray/operative findings

X-ray	Granulomatous mastoiditis		Osteolytic mastoiditis		Concomitant mastoiditis	
	n	%	n	%	n	%
Children (n = 95)						
Haziness with osteolysis	12	12	18	18	1	1
Haziness without osteolysis	31	32	18	18	8	10
Normal	3	4	2	3	2	2
Total		48		39		13
Adults (n = 59)						
Haziness with osteolysis	4	7	5	9	1	2
Haziness without osteolysis	31	52	11	19	0	
Normal	3	5	2	3	2	3
Total		64		31		5

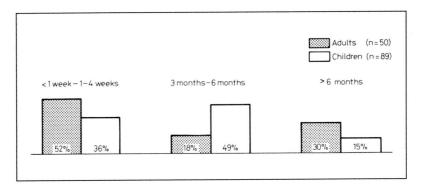

Fig. 2. Time interval between onset of otitis media and manifestation of complication.

Table VII. Predominant nonspecific symptoms of mastoiditis in children (n = 96)

	n	%
Dyspepsia	15	16
Infectious Anemia	3	3
Persistent fever	7	7
Recurrent bronchitis	2	2
Meningitis	3	3
Pathologic blood count and BSR	58	60

Discussion

The incidence of otogenic complications, due to oto-mastoiditis, is higher in adults (37%) than in children (10%). This finding is quite unexpected because of the overall incidence of otitis media is definitely higher in infants and children than in adolescents and adults. According to Stangerup and Tos [1986] the incidence is highest in the first year of life (22%), after which time it gradually decreases from 15% in the second to 2% in the eighth year. By the age of 9 years 75% of all the children have had at least one episode of otitis media. This statistic supports the view that the development of general and local immunodefense mechanisms in the upper respiratory tract and the middle ear cleft is achieved by reaching adolescence. Kalm [1986] has observed in children affected with recurrent otitis media very low antibody concentrations, compared with healthy children. In the following, however, he was able to demonstrate a gradual increase to equal level in adulthood. This finding indicates a selective delay of immunological maturation within the recurrent otitis media group. However, if in a later period of life these defence mechanisms break down it seems that the immunodefense mechanisms located in the muco-periosteum of the middle ear compartments are more often severely impaired than general immunological reactions. This might explain why in the group of adults the risk of a local complication such as labyrinthitis (6/24 cases) or facial palsy (8/24 cases) is much higher than the risk of an intracranial complication such as meningitis or thrombosis of the lateral sinus. In our group of children, however, intracranial complications occur as frequently as local complications. This phenomenon may be explained by the fact that during this early period of life immunodefense mechanisms are not yet fully developed and virulent infections will spread much more easily along preformed routes into the endocranium. This view is supported by the observation that in our material *H. influenzae* meningitis occurred only during early childhood. In 1 infant and in 1 child (2 years) *H. influenzae* meningitis developed insidiously 3–4 weeks after the onset of an acute otitis media under antibiotic treatment. This observation brings up the problem of occult or silent otitis media. We agree with Paparella et al. [1986] that *silent otitis media associated with* H. influenzae *meningitis* '... seems to suggest a possible cause and effect relationship... It is possible that the trend towards conservative management of acute otitis media may have played a role in these children in masking the presence of pathological otitis media and therefore may have quietly predisposed to ... influenzae meningitis.'

The most important difference between our 2 age groups concerns the interval between the onset and treatment of an otitis media and the clinical manifestation of an oto-mastoiditis and its complications.

In our group of children mastoiditis incidence reaches its highest peak between the third and the sixth month after the onset of otitis media symptoms. In the group of adults, however, the highest peak of incidence is observed between the first and fourth week after the beginning of acute otitis media signs (difference statistically significant: $p < 0.01 > 0.001$).

We have tried to explain this phenomenon in a previous publication [Pfaltz and Griesemer, 1984] by the fact that at present a majority of pediatricians are convinced that they can cure any case of acute mastoiditis by long-term conservative therapy (early myringotomy and appropriate intravenous administration of antibiotics). They seem to be unaware of the fact that antibiotics have not only reduced the incidence of otogenic complications but also modified their symptoms. The insidious onset and relative rarity of these conditions means that they are often unrecognized until too late [Cheesman, 1979]. Hawkins et al. [1983] have pointed out quite recently that children who have been admitted with meningitis secondary to acute otitis media showed varying degrees of clouding on mastoid radiographs, but none of them had physical findings of acute mastoiditis. Antibiotic therapy has therefore definitely altered the course of the disease. In our series of mastoiditis in children and infants we found a *high incidence of nonspecific symptoms,* indicating a severe general infection, whereas characteristic or specific physical signs of otitis media and mastoiditis were either mild or even completely missing.

It is well known that acute otitis media is a common condition in infants but only rarely is the general physician's attention drawn to the ears because otorrhea is mostly a late symptom and the other cardinal symptoms, such as earache and deafness, cannot be noticed. Moreover, otoscopic findings may be rather discrete. For those reasons, antibiotic treatment is often started too late, when the infection has already spread into the antrum and the adjacent cell groups of the mastoid process, where it can no longer be safely controlled. Prellner and Rydell [1985] have recently carried out a study on the influence of antibiotic treatment on the bacterial spectrum in acute mastoiditis. From their results they conclude that purulent secretion in the mastoid cells is often sterilized by antibiotics, even when treatment has been of rather short duration. These data strongly indicate that antibiotic treatment even of short duration is of a major importance for the bacterial flora obtained in acute mastoiditis. On the other hand, it also shows that the *bacterial infection* of the middle ear cleft but not the *inflammatory process* within the pneumatic system of the mastoid process has been eradicated. Under antibiotic treatment an *occult or silent mastoiditis* is gradually developing followed eventually by an intracranial complication.

These cases of so called *masked mastoiditis* may eventually be due to inadequate antibiotic therapy; but the clinical entity of masked mastoiditis was already known in the pre-antibiotic era [Marx, 1947; Goodhill, 1979]. These cases were and still are particularly dangerous because during the stage of a latent rarefying osteitis, the inflammatory process will only occasionally break through the cortex of the mastoid but more often into the endocranium, the lateral sinus, either by continuity or more often by following preformed pathways. Therefore, antibiotics do not seem to have entirely changed the course of mastoiditis because the incidence of local and even endocranial otogenic complications is still rather high, even under the favorable socioeconomic conditions existing in Western Europe. But antibiotics have changed the course of otitis media, which may turn into a *silent otitis media,* masking its symptoms, predisposing to the development of a *masked or occult mastoiditis* which will end up eventually in an *intracranial complication.*

Conclusions

(1) *Antibiotics* have not only reduced the incidence of otogenic complications *but also* modified their symptoms, particularly in children.

(2) *Antibiotics* may eradicate the infection within the middle ear cleft, *but not* always stop the inflammatory process within the mastoid.

(3) In *early childhood* the *prevalent symptoms* leading to the diagnosis of otomastoiditis are *unspecific* in the majority of cases, whereas in *adults* they are *entirely specific.*

(4) In *adults* mastoiditis *incidence* reaches its highest peak 1–4 weeks, in *infants and children* 3–6 months after the onset of an otitis media. This is the most dangerous period with respect to the silent development of an intracranial complication, due to an occult mastoiditis.

(5) Depending on the *virulence* and the *resistance* of the infectious agent, the integrity of the general and the local mucoperiosteal *immuno-defence-mechanisms, silent otitis media* may develop, leading to a *masked mastoiditis,* which can result in a local, extracranial or a general intracranial complication.

References

Cheesman, A.D.: Ear infections; in Maran, Stell, Clinical otolaryngology, pp. 171–181 (Blackwell, Oxford 1979).

Ginsburg, C.M.; Rudoy, R.; Nelson, J.D.: Acute mastoiditis in infants and children. Clin. Pediat. *19:* 549–553 (1980).

Goodhill, V.: Ear diseases, deafness and dizziness, pp. 294–306 (Harper & Row, New York 1979).

Hawkins, D.B.; Dru, D.; House, J.W.; Clark, R.W.: Acute mastoiditis in children. A review of 54 cases. Laryngoscope *93:* 568–572 (1983).

Kalm, O.: Recurrent acute otitis media. Immunological and clinical aspects; thesis, University of Lund (Infotryck, Malmö 1986).

Marx, H.: Kurzes Handbuch der Ohrenheilkunde, 2nd ed., pp. 1–266 (Fischer, Jena 1947).

Palva, T.; Virtanen, H.; Mäkinen, J.: Acute and latent mastoiditis in children. J. Lar. Otol. *99:* 127–136 (1985).

Paparella, M.M.; Goycoolea, M.; Bassiouni, M.; Kontroupas, S.: Silent otitis media. Clinical applications. Laryngoscope *96:* 978–985 (1986).

Pfaltz, C.R.; Griesemer, C.: Complications of acute middle ear infections. Ann. Otol. Rhinol. Lar. *93:* suppl. 112, pp. 133–136 (1984).

Prellner, K.; Rydell, R.: Acute mastoiditis. Influence of antibiotic treatment on the bacterial spectrum. Acta oto-lar. *99:* 293–297 (1985).

Samuel, J.; Fernandes, C.M.C.; Steinberg, J.L.: Intracranial otogenic complications. A persisting problem. Laryngoscope *96:* 272–278 (1986).

Scheydt, P.C.; Kavanagh, J.F.: Common terminology for conditions of the middle ear; in Kavanagh, Otitis media and child development, p. XV (Parkton-Maryland-York Press, London 1986).

Schuknecht, H.Г.: Pathology of the ear, p. 220 (Harvard University Press, Cambridge 1974).

Stangerup, S.E.; Tos, M.: Epidemiology of acute suppurative otitis media. Am. J. Otolar. *7:* 47–54 (1986).

Stangerup, S.E.; Tos, M.: Etiological role of acute suppurative otitis media in chronic secretory otitis. Am. J. Otolar. *6:* 126–131 (1985).

Prof. Dr. C.R. Pfaltz, Department of ORL, University Hospital Basel,
CH–4031 Basel (Switzerland)

Adv. Oto-Rhino-Laryng., vol. 40, pp. 81–88 (Karger, Basel 1988)

Tonsils and Adenoids

Their Relation to Secretory Otitis media

A. Richard Maw

Consultant Otolaryngologist, Royal Hospital for Sick Children and
Bristol Royal Infirmary, Bristol, UK

Introduction

Previous reports have demonstrated clearance of effusions in 40 per cent of children suffering with established secretory otitis media (SOM) or glue ear 12 months after treatment by adenoidectomy or adeno-tonsillectomy [1]. Commensurate impedance change from flat non-peaked type B curves to peaked A, C1 or C2 curves have also been shown. Furthermore, a significant puretone audiometric hearing gain has been demonstrated. Six months post-operatively, the beneficial effects were all more marked, though not statistically significant, in the adeno-tonsillectomy group compared with the adenoidectomy group. However, after 12 months the trend reversed in favour of adenoidectomy. Thus, it appeared that tonsillectomy conferred no extra long-term benefit in the treatment of SOM compared with adenoidectomy alone. Consequently, random allocation for tonsillectomy in combination with adenoidectomy was discontinued after 150 cases had been evaluated. The present report re-evaluates the previous data with 42 additional cases, again satisfying the same entry criteria but allocated randomly into either adenoidectomy or no surgery groups. As before in all cases the effusions were bilateral. A myringotomy and ventilation tube insertion was performed at random in one ear. The contralateral ear was not submitted to any surgery, but was re-examined for clearance of the effusion, impedance change and puretone audiometric hearing gain. The results of these three parameters are presented 12, 24 and 36 months following surgery. The design of the study permits evaluation of the effects of adenoidectomy, adeno-tonsillectomy, and ventilation tube insertion separately. It also demonstrates the natural history of the untreated condition in these children.

Materials and Methods

Approval for the study was obtained from the District Ethical Committee. There were five absolute criteria for entry. Firstly, the age range was between 2 and 9 years. Secondly, complaint or report of persistent subjective hearing loss was a mandatory requirement. Thirdly, pneumatic otoscopy by a validated observer confirmed bilateral middle ear effusions. Fourthly impedance studies showed either type B, C1 or C2 curves and in no case was a type A curve present. Fifthly where possible puretone audiometry showed in excess of 25 dB hearing loss in each ear at one or more frequencies. All of the criteria were satisfied at the first consultation and again at the second and third examinations, 6 and 12 weeks later. Between July 1979 and January 1984 322 children entered the study. For reasons previously reported [1] but mainly because the effusion resolved in one or both ears, 159 children were excluded at the first or second appointments. Surgery was carried out by allocation at random into three groups. Adeno-tonsillectomy (47 cases), adenoidectomy (47 cases) no surgery (56 cases). Thirteen cases were excluded at operation. Between January 1984 and April 1986 a further 84 cases satisfying the same criteria entered the study. At the second or third appointment 42 were excluded and 42 were therefore allocated at random into adenoidectomy and no-surgery groups. Thus increasing the numbers in these groups to 70 and 75, respectively. The cases were re-examined 1, 2 and 3 years after operation. Similar otoscopic examination was made by the same observer without knowledge of the operative grouping. Identical impedance and audiometric studies were performed. At each follow-up time not all of the children attended and some would not co-operate with the investigations. In some cases where there was persistence of fluid in the unoperated ear and where the ventilation tube in the operated ear had extruded with reaccumulation of an effusion, recurrence of significant hearing difficulty necessitated re-insertion of a tube. This was always into the previously operated ear.

Results

Examination of the unoperated ear in the three groups allows assessment of the effects of adeno-tonsillectomy and adenoidectomy in isolation. It also allows assessment of the effects of ventilation tube insertion (and re-insertion) alone. The unoperated ear in the no-surgery group reflects the natural history of the untreated condition.

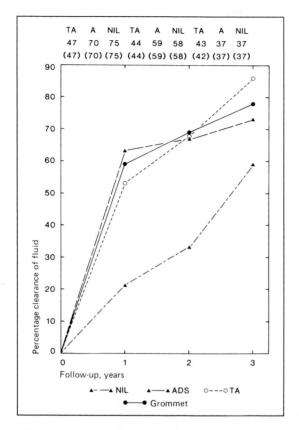

Fig. 1. Percentage clearance of fluid in the unoperated ear in the three groups and the clearance in the ear treated with a ventilation tube.

Clearance of Effusion

Figure 1 shows the percentage clearance of fluid in the unoperated ear in the three groups and also the clearance in the ear treated with a ventilation tube. The absolute numbers of children in the three groups are shown, together with the actual numbers of children attending and co-operating with the investigations at each time (number in parentheses). Chi-squared analysis shows a highly significant clearance of effusion in the unoperated ear of the three groups treated surgically at both 1 and 2 years, compared with the ear not submitted to any treatment. At 3 years there is a significant clearance as a result of adeno-tonsillectomy, but only a trend in the ears treated by adenoidectomy or tube insertion.

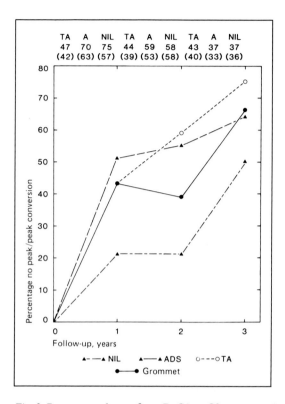

Fig. 2. Percentage change from B, C1 or C2 curves to A, C1 or C2 curves.

Impedance Change

The pre-operative impedance curves were type B in 98% of cases. C1 or C2 curves were present in 2%. Figure 2 shows the percentage change from B, C1 or C2 curves to A, C1 or C2 curves. There is a significant difference between the untreated ear and those treated by adeno-tonsillectomy at 1, 2 and 3 years. There is a significant improvement in the adenoidectomy group, but only 2 years following surgery.

Change in Mean Hearing Thresholds

In most cases puretone audiometric thresholds were estimated at six frequencies. In younger children only three frequencies were obtained and in a few very young children a free-field assessment was made. The mean of the pre-operative thresholds was greater than 30 dB in all ears in all

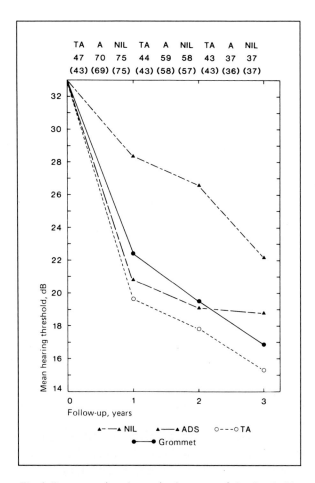

Fig. 3. Post-operative change in the mean of the thresholds.

groups. The post-operative change in the mean of the thresholds is shown in figure 3. Compared with the unoperated ear in the no-surgery group analysis of variants and paired t tests show a significant hearing gain at each follow-up time as a result of the three surgical procedures.

Ventilation Tube Re-Insertion

During the 3-year period recurrence of significant subjective hearing loss necessitated re-insertion of ventilation tubes. In some cases re-insertion was required on more than one occasion following repeated extrusion.

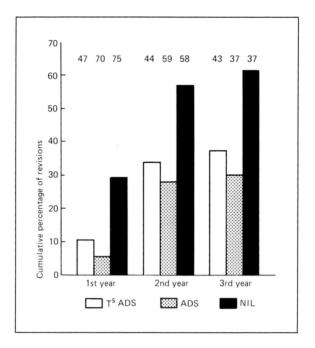

Fig. 4. Cumulative percentage of re-insertions in the three groups at each follow-up time.

Figure 4 shows the cumulative percentage of re-insertions in the three groups at each follow-up time. The difference between the two surgical groups and the no-treatment group is significant at each time.

Discussion

In most centres tonsillectomy in combination with adenoidectomy is less frequently recommended than adenoidectomy alone for treatment of SOM. Few of the previously reported studies investigate adenoidectomy alone. Most report the effect of adenoidectomy in combination with insertion of a ventilation tube [2, 3]. The present investigation allows each of these surgical procedures to be assessed in isolation. We have demonstrated the effect of the operations on clearance of effusion judged by pneumatic otoscopy. There is seen to be a reasonable correlation between the results of this assessment and the change in impedance measurements. As expected the latter change from flat to peaked curves less rapidly than the changes seen on otoscopy. Finally, all three of the operative procedures produced significant hearing gain which continues to improve as follow-up progresses.

By each parameter of assessment there is a slow but steady improvement in the state of the unoperated ear in the no-surgery group reflecting spontaneous improvement in Eustachian tube function and the clearance of the effusion as the child grows older. However, when on average these children would be aged 8.25 years effusions are still present in 40%, impedance conversion has not taken place in 50% and there is still a mean hearing loss of 22 dB.

In the ears treated by insertion of a ventilation tube, re-insertion is required twice as frequently if a tube is used alone, than if it is combined with adenoidectomy or adeno-tonsillectomy. Only if used in isolation was there a need to re-insert a ventilation tube on as many as four occasions during this period of time.

Other data from this study has shown a significant development of tympano-sclerosis in ears treated by tube insertion [4]. 40% of cases were affected by some degree of sclerosis after 1 year and 70% after 2 years. In the unoperated ear tympano-sclerosis of a significant degree was never found. There was seen to be progression of the sclerotic change through the tympanic membrane as time passed. We have found no significant difference in audiometric thresholds in operated ears 3 years after ventilation tube insertion. However, unreported data shows poorer hearing thresholds in children with more extensive tympano-sclerosis five years after tube insertion ($p < 0.05$).

Summary and Conclusions

This study demonstrates a significant resolution of effusions which is maintained for at least 3 years. Improvement results both from adenoidectomy alone and in combination with tonsillectomy. Significant audiometric hearing gain also occurs. There is a slight but statistically insignificant trend in favour of the combined operation, compared with adenoidectomy alone. Similar improvements can be achieved by use of a ventilation tube. But re-insertion is required twice as frequently with a tube alone than in cases where it is combined with adenoidectomy or adeno-tonsillectomy.

The relative rates for mortality and morbidity of ventilation tube alone, adenoidectomy or adeno-tonsillectomy are well recognised. Taking these into account and considering the findings of this study there would seem to be little additional benefit from combination of tonsillectomy with adenoidectomy compared with adenoidectomy alone. The necessity for a second or subsequent anaesthetic in cases treated with a tube alone must also be considered. These results give some support to the suggestion that the treatment of choice for established bilateral SOM may be adenoidectomy in selected cases, combined with unilateral insertion of a ventilation tube. The latter procedure effects immediate but short-lived hearing gain. Unilateral compared with bilateral insertion reduces the overall complication rate due to the tube by 50%. The former procedure effects sustained improvement which persists following extrusion of the tube. Further prospective studies are required to predict more precisely those cases in which adenoidectomy should be recommended.

References

1   Maw, A.R.; Herod, F.: Otoscopic, impedance and audiometric findings in glue ear treated by adenoidectomy and tonsillectomy. A prospective randomized study. Lancet *i:* 1399–1402 (1986).
2   Black, N.; Crowther, J.; Freeland, A.: The effectiveness of adenoidectomy in the treatment of glue ear. A randomized controlled trial. Clin. Otolar. *11:* 149–155 (1986).
3   Widemar, L.; Svensson, C.; Rynell-Dagoo, B.; Schiratzkj, H.: The effect of adenoidectomy on secretory otitis media. A two-year controlled prospective study. Clin. Otolar. *10:* 345–350 (1985).
4   Slack, R.W.T.; Maw, A.R.; Capper, J.W.R.; Kelly, S.: A prospective study of tympanosclerosis developing after grommet insertion. J. Lar. Otol. *98:* 771–774 (1984).

A. Richard Maw, M.S., FRCS, Consultant Otolaryngologist,
Royal Hospital for Sick Children and Bristol Royal Infirmary, Bristol (UK)

Adv. Oto-Rhino-Laryng., vol. 40, pp. 89–98 (Karger, Basel 1988)

Secretory Otitis media: What Effects on Children's Development?

Jack L. Paradise

Departments of Pediatrics and Community Medicine of the University of Pittsburgh School of Medicine and the Ambulatory Care Center of the Children's Hospital of Pittsburgh, Pittsburgh, Pa., USA

Prevalence of Secretory Otitis media

Probably the most prevalent physical illness among western-world infants and young children is secretory otitis media. A survey conducted some years ago during the winter months in Washington, D.C. showed that 20–30% of presumably healthy children in the younger age groups had active middle-ear inflammation [1]. This impressive prevalence weighs heavily in current concern among health professionals about possible effects of secretory otitis media early in life on later speech, language, cognitive, intellectual, and emotional development [2, 3].

The Question: Effects of Early Otitis on Later Development

The question is *not* whether adverse developmental effects can result from otitis media which persists unremittingly, accompanied by conductive hearing loss, into the early school-age years. Most critical observers would readily agree that such long-standing hearing loss is likely to be developmentally harmful. Rather, the question is whether otitis with hearing loss that resolves within the first one, two, or three years of life nonetheless leaves in its wake enduring, and perhaps irreparable, damage to presumably critical developmental processes which had been occurring during presumably critical or sensitive periods.

The question borrows a concept from studies in laboratory animals. These studies point to critical or sensitive periods in the development of the animals' brains, during which sensory deprivation can apparently result in permanent functional, and even structural, derangements [2]. The hypothesized analogous deficits in children may be thought of as 'developmental scars' as a result of early auditory 'deprivation' [4]. This concept has found expression in a growing number of publications in both professional and lay literature [2, 3, 5].

Implications of the Question

The possibility that late developmental effects result from early otitis clearly has enormous practical and public health importance, and major implications regarding health-care practices. If, during infancy and early childhood, the variable hearing impairment that accompanies middle-ear effusion constitutes – even after relatively short periods - a risk factor in regard to any aspect of development, aggressive treatment measures would seem appropriate, even if costly and not wholly risk-free, as in the case of tympanostomy-tube placement. If, on the other hand, developmental effects do not result from these hearing impairments, or if effects do result but disappear once middle-ear effusions resolve, watchful waiting rather than prompt surgical intervention would constitute the more prudent course to follow.

Studies Supporting a Relationship

What is the nature of the evidence that bears on this question? The prototypical study was reported by Holm and Kunze [6] in 1969. These investigators compared two groups of school-aged children – an experimental group who as infants and young children had had a great deal of otitis media that subsequently resolved, and a control group not known ever to have had middle-ear problems. The two groups were matched for age, sex, and socioeconomic status, and were given a series of 12 developmental tests involving IQ, speech, and language. At the time of testing none of the children showed substantial hearing loss. For each of the 12 tests the mean score was higher for the control children, and for many of the tests, the difference between the two groups reached statistical significance.

The authors of this report recognized the limitations of their study, and drew no sweeping conclusions. They pointed out merely that their results *suggested* that middle-ear disease early in life *might* have long-term adverse developmental consequences. Later authors, however, in referring to this study, have stated without qualification that the study demonstrated that such adverse consequences do indeed develop [2].

There followed a series of reports of ten additional studies, most retrospective in nature, that came to similar conclusions – namely, that there was indeed a relationship between early otitis media and later developmental handicaps [7–16].

Evaluating Studies: Three Main Issues

The question of such a relationship can be seen on close examination to contain three elements: (1) Is there indeed an association between early otitis media and later developmental impairment? (2) If an association exists, is it cause-and-effect in nature? (3) If developmental impairments do result from early otitis media, are the impairments irreversible?

Detailed analyses concerning the various reported studies, with specific reference to each of these three issues, have previously been advanced [2, 5, 17]. I shall summarize the salient problems, as I view them, regarding study design, methodology, and interpretation of data.

Is There a Real Association?

First, the question whether the studies indeed demonstrate that an association exists between early otitis and developmental impairment. In addressing this question the studies collectively pose a wide range of problems affecting the validity of their findings. The problems may be grouped into nine categories. Not every one of the eleven studies was problematic in each of the nine categories, but all were problematic in most.

Nonrepresentativeness

The first problem was that the population groups from whom subjects were selected were, in most instances, not representative. Many of the studies involved economically or culturally deprived children, or children referred for evaluation because of some type of identified disability or underachievement.

Selection Bias

The second problem involves the risk of selection bias. Parents volunteering or consenting to have their children participate in the studies are likely to have differed from the parents of nonparticipating children in complex ways, involving characteristics with potentially important bearing on study outcomes. For example, participation might have been fostered, on the one hand, by concern that a child actually had a speech or language problem, or, on the other hand, by personal attributes, such as interest, organization, cooperativeness, and curiosity, likely to have promoted the development of superior speech and language. Unless parental characteristics such as these were distributed equally between the experimental and control groups, they could have had substantial potential for confounding the results.

Inadequate Ascertainment Concerning Otitis media

Third is the problem of inadequate ascertainment. In most of the studies, determination of the presence or absence of otitis media during early life was based on either parental recall, or a retrospective review of available medical records, or both. Where recall was the basis, episodes of otitis might have been recalled better by parents whose children had language or learning problems than by parents whose children did not have such problems. Where records provided the basis, ascertainment might have been compromised by the difficulty of determining accurately the presence or absence of middle-ear effusion, especially in infants and young children, and by possible detection bias introduced by variability in the frequency with which subjects had been examined.

No Hearing Data

The fourth problem is that none of the studies provided data concerning actual hearing acuity during early life. Of critical importance would have been whether hearing loss was long-standing or transient; bilateral or unilateral; and severe, moderate, or mild.

Questionable Matching

The fifth problem concerns the difficulty of achieving adequate matching of experimental and control subjects regarding the many variables capable of affecting developmental outcome, such as socioeconomic status, degree and character of social and intellectual stimulation, and quality of parenting.

Persistently Impaired Hearing

The sixth problem concerns the requirement that if one wishes to test the effects of hearing loss that was limited to the first few years of life, then hearing at the time of developmental testing should be normal. Yet in most of the studies, at the time the subjects received developmental testing, hearing acuity either was somewhat poorer in the experimental group than in the control group, or was not reported for either group.

Questionable Validity of Test Results

The seventh problem is that, in many of the studies, the validity of the developmental test results was uncertain, for one or more of several reasons. The individuals performing the developmental testing may not have been blinded to which of the children were the experimental subjects and which the controls. Moreover, most reports provided no information regarding either the number of examiners administering the developmental tests, the nature of their qualifications, the conditions of testing, or the degree of consistency in the order of test presentation. Finally, the developmental test instruments employed may not have been age-appropriate, and in some instances their reliability and validity had not been previously established.

Summary Statistics Rather than Data

The eighth problem is that reported results often were limited to a presentation of summary statistics, rather than of actual data in sufficient detail to permit independent analysis. For example, many reports, rather than providing frequency distributions, ranges, or medians of test scores, provided only means, which could have been influenced by extreme individual values, and standard deviations, which might not have adequately characterized the scores' distributions [18].

Selective Emphasis of Positive Findings

And, finally, the ninth problem is that in some of the studies, the authors focused on, or based conclusions on, only certain of their findings, ignoring other findings that failed to support, or even argued against, their hypotheses.

If an Association Exists, Is It Causal?

Even if we put aside these various problems of design and methodology, and for the sake of discussion accept that the first issue is settled and that an association between early otitis and later developmental handicaps does exist, we then come to the second issue, namely, whether such an association might be causal in nature. Here the concept faces further obstacles, since it is possible to imagine quite a few factors that might predispose *both* to susceptibility to otitis media on the one hand, *and* to substandard performance or developmental tests on the other.

Examples of such possible commonly underlying factors include adverse antenatal and perinatal events; any central nervous system disorder that might be associated with muscular hypotonia and might therefore affect Eustachian tube function adversely; and potentially adverse factors involving general health and function, such as recurrent or chronic respiratory infection, or respiratory or other types of allergy. Under such circumstances otitis media might be a *marker* of the developmentally vulnerable child rather than the *cause* of the child's vulnerability.

If Impairments Develop, Are They Irreversible?

Lastly, setting aside for a moment doubts about both association and causality, and assuming that otitis might indeed result directly in developmental impairments, we come to the third issue, namely, what evidence exists that such impairments would be irreversible?

Data bearing on this question are scant. However, in two reported studies of children with low developmental scores and histories of early otitis media, the developmental scores improved with increasing age [7, 19].

Studies Not Supporting a Relationship

In contrast to the studies purporting to show that early otitis results in later development impairment, a largely more recent group of studies have been reported in which associations between early otitis media and later developmental impairment were not found [20–27]. The design, the quality, and the degree of conclusiveness of these negative studies have been variable. Most suffer from many of the same shortcomings ascribed to the studies with positive findings. In addition, most of the studies lack consideration of type II error, that is, the risk that the study failed to detect an association that was actually present. While some of these negative studies seem convincing in some respects, neither individually nor collectively can they be considered to have conclusively *disproven* a relationship between early otitis and later developmental impairment. Nonetheless I would like to review certain data from one of the studies [26] – performed at our center in Pittsburgh – that I believe overcame many of the difficulties of previously reported studies.

Pittsburgh Study of Children with Cleft Palate

In designing the study we took advantage of two phenomena: first, that in infants and young children with cleft palate, otitis media with effusion is virtually universal, and second, that there existed in Pittsburgh two centers for treatment of cleft palate – a University Center and a Hospital Center – that for many years had similar patient populations and maintained apparently uniform approaches to management, except regarding persistent otitis media during early life. At the University Center, patients had received myringotomy with placement of tympanostomy tubes early in infancy, followed by close monitoring and an aggressive treatment program to maintain middle-ear ventilation. At the Hospital Center, most patients had received initial myringotomy later in childhood or not at all, and these patients had therefore presumably had continuous middle-ear effusion throughout most or all of the first few years of life. To determine whether these differences between University Center and Hospital Center patients in management, and in middle-ear status in early life, would be reflected at later ages by differences in developmental status, we compared 24 matched pairs of school-aged children, each pair consisting of one child from each center whose care had been provided at that center from early infancy.

The subjects were matched for cleft type, sex, age, socioeconomic status, and birth order. They then received a series of examinations from professionals unaware of which center the children had been enrolled in.

In the University Center group, 16 of the 24 subjects had received myringotomy with tube placement by 3 months of age, and the remaining 8 by 1 year of age. In contrast, in the Hospital Center group, only 1 subject had received tube placement by 3 months of age, and only 3 additional subjects by 1 year of age. Thirteen of the 24 Hospital Center subjects received tube placement only after 36 months of age, and 2 never received the operation. After about 3 years of age, otologic management in the

University and Hospital groups were comparable, with many children in both groups receiving one or more subsequent tube-placement procedures.

At 5–11 years of age the children in the two groups were very similar otoscopically and also very similar tympanometrically. Hearing thresholds were slightly higher in the Hospital Center group, but the differences between the two groups were small and probably unimportant clinically. The two groups differed substantially in the competence of their speech, as measured by a 162-item test of consonant articulation. The proportion of children with less than 80% correct responses was 17% in the University Center group, compared with 54% in the Hospital Center group (p < 0.05). Comparison of the two groups regarding verbal, performance, and full-scale IQ showed no differences favoring either group, and the same was true regarding several tests of social and emotional development.

Summarizing the results, early tube placement in the University Center group appeared to result, at later ages, in slightly better hearing and substantially better articulation than in the Hospital Center group, but there were no detectable differences between the two groups in cognitive, linguistic, or social and emotional development.

Keeping in mind that few infants and young children in the general population have middle-ear effusion as unremittingly as do infants and young children with cleft palate, I believe that this study's positive and negative findings, respectively, permit the following tentative conclusions and inferences:

(1) Long, uninterrupted periods (for example, 1 year or longer) of bilateral secretory otitis media in infancy and early childhood may result in residual hearing impairment of mild degree, and in impairment of consonant articulation.

(2) Other developmental areas – namely cognitive, language, and psychosocial development – seem unlikely to be adversely affected on a long-term basis.

(3) Short periods – for example, 3–4 months – of middle-ear effusion are probably harmless developmentally.

I must emphasize, however, the necessarily tentative nature of conclusions that are based on a single study of a specific subgroup of children.

North Carolina Study

A more recent, carefully conducted study in a group of socioeconomically deprived children [27] gave similarly negative results regarding the effects of early otitis media on later verbal and academic functions. However, small but important effects may have gone undetected in that study because of limited sample size.

Importance of Answering the Question

I have attempted to demonstrate that the question of a relationship between otitis media early in life and later developmental status must be considered largely unsettled. I hope that I have been able to summarize adequately the complexity of the question, and the potential pitfalls in studying it. Because the question involves so many children – literally millions – and because the health issues are so important, it is urgent that research in this area continues until satisfactory answers have been found.

References

1   Kessner, D.M.; Snow, C.K.; Singer, J.: Assessment of medical care for children: contrasts in health status, pp. 38–54 (Institute of Medicine, National Academy of Sciences, Washington 1974).
2   Paradise, J.L.: Otitis media during early life; how hazardous to development? A critical review of the evidence. Pediatrics, Springfield 68: 869–873 (1981).
3   Bluestone, C.D.; Klein, J.O.; Paradise, J.L.: Workshop on effects of otitis media on the child. Pediatrics, Springfield 71: 639–652 (1983).
4   Paradise, J.L.: Editorial retrospective; tympanometry. New Engl. J. Med. 307: 1074–1076 (1982).
5   Paradise, J.L.; Rogers, K.D.: On otitis media, child development, and tympanostomy tubes: New answers or old questions? Pediatrics, Springfield 77: 86–92 (1986).
6   Holm, V.A.; Kunze, L.H.: Effect of chronic otitis media on language and speech development. Pediatrics, Springfield 43: 833–839 (1969).
7   Needleman, H.: Effects of hearing loss from early recurrent otitis media on speech and language development; in Jaffe, Hearing loss in children, pp. 640–649 (University Park Press, Baltimore 1977).
8   Howie, V.M.: Acute and recurrent otitis media; in Jaffe, Hearing loss in children, pp. 421–429 (University Park Press, Baltimore 1977).
9   Zinkus, P.W.; Gottlieb, M.I.; Schapiro, M.: Developmental and psychoeducational sequelae of chronic otitis media. Am. J. Dis. Child. 132: 1100–1104 (1977).
10 Gottlieb, M.I.; Zinkus, P.W.; Thompson, A.: Chronic middle ear disease and auditory perceptual deficits, is there a link? Clin. Pediat. 18: 725–732 (1979).
11 Howie, V.M.; Jensen, N.J.; Fleming, J.W.; Peeler, M.B.; Meigs, S.: The effect of early onset of otitis media on educational achievement. Int. J. pediat. Otorhinolar. 1: 151–155 (1979).

12   Kessler, M.E.; Randolph, K.: The effects of early middle ear disease on the auditory
     abilities of third grade children. J. Acad. rehab. Audiol. *12:* 6–20 (1979).
13   Zinkus, P.W.; Gottlieb, M.I.: Patterns of perceptual and academic deficits related to
     early chronic otitis media. Pediatrics, Springfield *66:* 246–253 (1980).
14   Brandes, P.J.; Ehinger, D.M.: The effects of middle ear pathology on auditory per-
     ception and academic achievement. J. Speech Hear Dis. *46:* 250–257 (1981).
15   Sak, R.J.; Ruben, R.J.: Recurrent middle ear effusion in childhood; implication of
     temporary auditory deprivation for language and learning. Ann. Otol. Rhinol. Lar.
     90: 546–551 (1981).
16   Teele, D.W.; Klein, J.O.; Rosner, B.A.: Otitis media with effusion during the first
     three years of life and development of speech and language. Pediatrics, Springfield
     74: 282–287 (1984).
17   Paradise, J.L.: Long-term effects of short-term hearing loss – menace or myth?
     Workshop on the effects of otitis media on the child. Pediatrics, Springfield *71:*
     647–648 (1983).
18   Fletcher, R.H.; Fletcher, S.W.; Wagner, E.H.: Clinical epidemiology, pp. 26–31
     (Williams & Williams, Baltimore 1982).
19   Dalzell, J.; Owrid, H.L.: Children with conductive deafness. A follow-up study. Br. J.
     Audiol. *10:* 87–90 (1976).
20   Bennett, F.C.; Ruuska, S.H.; Sherman, R.: Middle ear function in learning-disabled
     children. Pediatrics, Springfield *66:* 254–260 (1980).
21   Hoffman-Lawless, K.; Keith, R.W.; Cotton, R.T.: Auditory processing abilities in
     children with previous middle ear effusion. Ann. Otol. Rhinol. Lar. *90:* 543–545
     (1981).
22   Friel-Patti, S.; Finitzo-Hieber, T.; Conti, G.; et al.: Language delay in infants asso-
     ciated with middle ear disease and mild fluctuating hearing impairment. Pediat.
     infect. Dis. *1:* 104–109 (1982).
23   Lous, J.; Fiellau-Nikolajsen, M.: A 5-year prospective case-control study of the
     influence of early otitis media with effusion on reading achievement. Int. J. pediat.
     Otorhinolar. *8:* 19–30 (1984).
24   Allen, D.V.; Robinson, D.O.: Middle ear status and language development in pre-
     school children. ASHA, 1984, pp. 33–37.
25   Fischler, R.S.; Todd, N.W.; Feldman, C.M.: Otitis media and language performance
     in a cohort of Apache Indian children. Am. J. Dis. Child. *139:* 355–360 (1985).
26   Hubbard, T.W.; Paradise, J.L.; McWilliams, B.J.; Elster, B.A.; Taylor, F.H.: Conse-
     quences of unremitting middle ear disease in early life. Otologic, audiologic, and
     developmental findings in children with cleft palate. New Engl. J. Med. *312:* 1529–
     1534 (1985).
27   Roberts, J.E.; Sanyal, M.A.; Burchinal, M.R.; Collier, A.M.; Raney, C.T.; Hender-
     son, F.W.: Otitis media in early childhood and its relationship to later verbal and
     academic performance. Pediatrics, Springfield *78:* 423–430 (1986).

Jack L. Paradise, MD, Departments of Pediatrics and Community Medicine,
University of Pittsburgh School of Medicine, Children's Hospital of Pittsburgh,
One Children's Place, 3705 Fifth Avenue et DeSoto Street,
Pittsburgh, PA 15213 (USA)

Adv. Oto-Rhino-Laryng., vol. 40, pp. 99–109 (Karger, Basel 1988)

Management of Secretory Otitis media

State of the Art

Jack L. Paradise

Departments of Pediatrics and Community Medicine of the University of Pittsburgh School of Medicine and the Ambulatory Care Center of the Children's Hospital of Pittsburgh, Pittsburgh, Pa., USA

The Disease Process

As a disease continuum otitis media comprises two principal elements: infection, or suppurative otitis media; and presumably noninfective inflammation accompanied by effusion, or secretory otitis media [1]. Eardrum findings in these two main types of otitis media are often similar, and the two types are closely interrelated clinically: pus in the middle-ear cavity is transformed into, or replaced by, nonpurulent-appearing effusion; in turn, the presence of effusion predisposes to the development of renewed infection. These interrelationships blur, to some extent, the distinction between the two types, as does the fact that secretory effusions sometimes harbor pathogenic bacteria [2–5]. On the other hand, secretory otitis sometimes develops without any apparent infectious element, presumably as a consequence of impaired middle-ear ventilation. Despite the difficulties sometimes encountered in distinguishing sharply between suppurative and secretory otitis media, the distinction is useful conceptually, and is firmly embedded in both clinical practice [6–8] and clinical investigation [9–11].

Natural History

The goal of management is to alter natural history in a favorable direction. Unfortunately, the natural history of secretory otitis media has not yet been fully charted, despite a number of excellent studies [12–21], mainly by our Danish colleagues. Lacking in particular is information concerning that small subgroup of children in whom secretory otitis fails to resolve spontaneously within a few months, and in whom surgical intervention is rightly or wrongly undertaken.

Symptoms, and Possible Complications and Sequelae

Two reasons exist for treating secretory otitis media: to alleviate symptoms, and to reduce the occurrence of complications and sequelae. In infants and young children with secretory otitis, symptoms tend to be notable by their absence. Hearing impairment not only is variable [22, 23], but even when present, often tends to go unnoticed. Manifestations of hearing impairment, such as discomfiture, unresponsiveness, and disturbed behavior, often are attributed by parents to other causes.

The presumed complications and sequelae of secretory otitis media fall into four main categories. The first category consists of the heightened probability that in the presence of secretory otitis, new episodes of infection are more likely than otherwise to occur.

In the second category are various structural changes that may conceivably result if secretory otitis is long-standing. These changes include retraction pockets, adhesive otitis, tympanic membrane scarring, ossicular discontinuity, and cholesteatoma [16, 24]. It seems unclear, however, whether these changes can develop in the absence of superimposed middle-ear infection.

The third category of sequelae consists of possible inner-ear damage with resulting sensorineural hearing loss [25, 26]. And the fourth category comprises the various impairments of development that may conceivably be attributable to longstanding conductive hearing loss.

As discussed elsewhere [1, 27] most observers would agree that bilateral hearing loss that persists throughout infancy and early childhood might indeed affect adversely many aspects of development – speech, linguistic, cognitive, intellectual, and emotional. However, regarding the effects of hearing loss that is limited to the first few years of life, little of the evidence reported to date can withstand critical scrutiny. Based on currently available information, I believe that adverse effects are unlikely to result unless secretory otitis media is of at least 6 months' duration, and involves both ears, and is accompanied by significant hearing loss – however that might be defined. When all of these circumstances do obtain, developmental effects may indeed be possible, but they may be limited to impaired speech – specifically, impaired articulation – with other aspects of development remaining essentially undisturbed [28]. I hasten to emphasize, however, that the facts of this matter are simply not known.

Management Options

Against this background of uncertainty about both physical and developmental sequelae, we may now consider the various options available for treating secretory otitis media. These too may be classified in four categories: medical, mechanical, surgical, and skeptical.

The medical options comprise antimicrobials, antihistamines and decongestants, and steroids. The mechanical options include use of the Valsalva maneuver, politzerization, and catheterization of the eustachian tube. Of these, only politzerization seems a feasible alternative for young children. The surgical options include myringotomy with aspiration, myringotomy with tympanostomy-tube placement, adenoidectomy, adenotonsillectomy, and various combinations of these procedures. And the last of the treatment options is to simply do nothing but monitor the child, in order to be certain that the situation does not deteriorate or become unduly prolonged.

Lack of Efficacy of Decongestant-Antihistamines

We now have answers – some reasonably firm, some only tentative - to some of the questions concerning the efficacy of various available medical treatments. Our group in Pittsburgh has shown conclusively, I believe, in a trial involving 553 children, that decongestant-antihistamine combinations – which had long been a standard mode of treatment - are *not* efficacious in treating secretory otitis media. Our study showed that in children with unilateral effusion at entry, 33.8% who received decongestant-antihistamine were free of effusion at 4 weeks, compared with 37.5% of those who received placebo. Of those with bilateral effusion at entry, the proportions effusion-free at 4 weeks were 20.7% in the drug-treated group and 18.5% in the placebo-treated group [29].

Efficacy of Amoxicillin

More recently, in a similarly designed study focusing on amoxicillin as the principal treatment, we compared results in 474 children randomly assigned to receive either a combination of amoxicillin and decongestant-antihistamine, or a combination of amoxicillin and a placebo, or two placebos. Among children with unilateral effusion at entry, the rate of resolution at four weeks ranged from 40.7 to 45.1% in the amoxicillin-treated groups, compared with 23.3% in the group receiving only placebo. Among those with bilateral effusion at entry, the rates of resolution were substantially lower, but again there was a substantial difference favoring the amoxicillin-treated groups, in whom the rate of resolution ranged from 22.6 to 25.2%, compared with 10.6% in the placebo-treated group [30]. The results in this trial incidentally confirmed the findings of the earlier trial, in which we found no substantial difference in outcome between groups who received decongestant-antihistamine and groups who did not [29].

Since previous investigators also had found antimicrobials – in the form of sulfonamides - efficacious to some extent [31, 32], it seems reasonable to conclude that antimicrobial drugs have a legitimate role to play in the management of secretory otitis media. The degree of efficacy will undoubtedly vary, and will depend on a number of factors, including the nature of the population being treated, the duration of the disease process, and the drug being used.

Factors Affecting Outcome

It seems important to emphasize that in both the decongestant-antihistamine and the amoxicillin trials, outcomes not only were substantially better in children who entered with unilateral than with bilateral otitis, but also were better in children without upper respiratory infection than with upper respiratory infection at the endpoints of the trials. The latter finding is in keeping with a precept I have long held, along with others [33, 34], to the effect that middle-ear effusion is unlikely to resolve unless all traces of nasal or paranasal infection can be eradicated.

Corticosteroids

The literature contains a number of studies of the efficacy of corticosteroids in treating secretory otitis media. Two randomized, double-blind studies are of particular interest. In the first of these, treatment with both oral dexamethasone and with placebo proved equally disappointing, with cure in only 1 child of 26 receiving dexamethasone, and in only 2 of 23 receiving placebo. On the basis of these preliminary findings the trial was interrupted, since continued administration of steroid was not considered justifiable. However, the low overall response rate raises the question whether the children were refractory because of long-standing disease, or for other reasons, and leaves open the possibility that oral steroids might be effective in certain patients, perhaps in those with disease that is less well established.

The second trial of steroids involved children with primary or new episodes of secretory otitis, who were assigned to treatment with either beclomethasone nasal spray or placebo. After one month of treatment, 18% of the ears in drug-treated children compared with 20% of ears in placebo-treated children showed clearance of effusion as estimated tympanometrically. One month later, 35% of the ears in the placebo-treated group showed resolution, compared with 25% in the drug-treated group [35].

It seems reasonable to conclude that the use of steroids in secretory otitis media deserves further study, but does not appear promising.

Politzerization

I know of no well-designed study testing the efficacy of politzerization in children. Politzerization would seem an attractive option for older children, and deserves systematic investigation.

Myringotomy with or without Tympanostomy Tube Placement – Benefits and Risks

Myringotomy with or without the placement of tympanostomy tubes constitutes an appealingly direct approach to the problem of secretory otitis media. Myringotomy permits evacuation of the middle-ear cavity, but often is followed by prompt healing of the eardrum incision and reaccumulation of middle-ear effusion. The addition of a tympanostomy tube, on the other hand, offers the promise of sustained middle-ear ventilation for as long as the tube remains in place.

Offsetting the benefits afforded by tubes – aside from the risks of the procedure and the not inconsiderable cost – is a substantial number of complications and sequalae. Obviously, the function of the tube is negated if its lumen becomes obstructed, or if it becomes extruded prematurely, or dislocated into the middle-ear cavity. Secondary infection with otorrhea through the tube occurs relatively frequently, and may sometimes be resistant to treatment. Of greater concern to me as a pediatrician are the changes seen in the eardrum following tubal extrusion. These changes consist mainly of minor or major scarring, that is, tympanosclerosis, and of localized or diffuse atrophy that may be accompanied by retraction pockets or atelectasis or both [36–46]. Such changes appear to occur increasingly as periods of intubation lengthen [36, 38, 39]. Less commonly, perforation remains at the insertion site following extrusion, or cholesteatoma develops. In a number of reports the combined rate of occurrence of all such abnormalities, after periods ranging up to 8 years from the time of tube insertion, has varied from 32 to 60% [41].

The importance of these eardrum abnormalities, other than cholesteatoma, seems debatable. On the one hand, it must be acknowledged that their long-range consequences are not yet fully known: some might conceivably predispose to the development of more serious middle-ear disease later, or to increasing deterioration of hearing [41, 43]. On the other hand, it can be argued that (1) in most instances the eardrum abnormalities are not accompanied by significant impairment of hearing; (2) some of the changes may well have been due to the underlying disease rather than the tubes; and (3) had tubes not been used, the otologic results might have been worse [47].

Finally, nuisance-value factors such as the necessity to avoid the introduction of water into the middle-ear cavity, and the occasional complaint of hyperacusis, complete the list of untoward outcomes.

Recurrence of middle-ear effusion following the extrusion of tubes has not been studied systematically, but appears to develop in at least 20–40% of the cases. [48–50].

Preliminary Results of the Pittsburgh Study

Our group in Pittsburgh has attempted to evaluate the efficacy of myringotomy alone, and of myringotomy with tympanostomy-tube placement, in relation to nonsurgical management. All subjects had had persistent secretory otitis media for 2 months or longer, and had failed to respond to preliminary antimicrobial treatment. During the first year after entry, children who received tube insertion remained generally free of middle-ear disease, whereas most control subjects, and most of those who received myringotomy only, continued to show evidence of middle-ear effusion. Poor outcomes in the myringotomy-only group occurred most often in subjects whose duration of effusion at entry was either 6 months or longer, or unknown [51].

It seems possible that the subjects of this study constituted an adversely selected subgroup, because of long duration of illness or for other reasons, and that myringotomy without tube placement might offer more satisfactory results in children seen under ordinary circumstances of practice. In my own experience, many patients with duration of effusion in the range of three months have responded satisfactorily to myringotomy only, and have subsequently remained effusion-free.

Current Recommendations

Certainly, recommendations regarding the management of secretory otitis media must be based to a considerable extent on opinion. My own recommendations are as follows: All cases should receive a course of at least 10 days of appropriate antimicrobial treatment, and this should be repeated if persistent upper respiratory infection recurs before middle-ear effusion has resolved.

After 3 months of effusion, and provided that there is absolutely no otoscopic or tympanometric evidence of improvement, myringotomy with aspiration, but without tube placement, seems appropriate. However, should there have been any indication of improvement, further temporizing would be called for instead.

If, following myringotomy, secretory otitis should recur within 6 months, and should again remain persistent despite appropriate antimicrobial treatment, tube placement would then seem advisable.

In other types of cases, if it can be established that middle-ear effusion that has not responded to treatment has been present for at least 6 months, tube placement is probably preferable as the initial procedure.

I offer these recommendations only as general guidelines. One might reasonably delay intervention longer if otitis media is unilateral, or if hearing is near-normal, or if hot weather is imminent. Or one might reasonably intervene earlier in children with sensorineural hearing loss, cleft palate, or uncontrolled upper respiratory allergy.

Adenoidectomy with or without Tonsillectomy

As to the possible role of adenoidectomy or adenotonsillectomy in the management of secretory otitis media, we must distinguish between management of the presenting episode and prevention of future episodes. Relatively few controlled trials have been reported [52–62], and for a variety of reasons their results have been variable. Based on the collective results, and on current analyses from our own study [63], it seems apparent that under certain circumstances adenoidectomy may reduce the subsequent occurrence of secretory otitis. However, the reduction is limited in degree, and has been found only in selected subgroups who are by no means representative of the general population of children with secretory otitis media. Accordingly, I believe that the appropriate role of adenoidectomy remains to be clarified, and that caution is essential in relating currently available research findings to everyday practice.

In summary, the state of the art regarding the management of secretory otitis media has been slowly improving, but wholly satisfactory methods are not yet available, and current methods have yet to be fully evaluated.

References

1   Paradise, J.L.: Otitis media in infants and children. Pediatrics, Springfield 65: 917–943 (1980).
2   Senturia, B.H.; Gessert, C.F.; Carr, C.D.; et al.: Studies concerned with tubotympanitis. Ann. Otol. Rhinol. Lar. 67: 440–467 (1958).
3   Liu, Y.S.; Lang, R.; Lim, D.J.; Birck, H.G.: Microorganisms in chronic otitis media with effusion. Ann. Otol. Rhinol. Lar. 85: suppl. 25, pp. 245–249 (1976).
4   Healy, G.B.; Teele, D.W.: The microbiology of chronic middle-ear effusions in children. Laryngoscope 87: 1472–1475 (1977).
5   Riding, K.H.; Bluestone, C.D.; Michaels, R.H.; et al.: Microbiology of recurrent and chronic otitis media with effusion. J. Pediat. 93: 739–743 (1978):
6   Politzer, A.: A textbook of the diseases of the ear: 5th ed., pp. 300–308 (Lea & Febiger, Philadelphia).
7   Nelson, J.D.: Otitis media; in Vaughn, McKay, Nelson, Nelson textbook of pediatrics; 10th ed., pp. 952–955 (Saunders, Philadelphia 1975).
8   Lewin, E.B.: Middle-ear disease; in Hoekelman, Blatman, Brunell, Principles of pediatrics, pp. 1730–1737 (Mc-Graw Hill, New York 1978).
9   Paparella, M.M.; Bluestone, C.D.; Arnold, W.; et al.: Panel 1A: Definition and classification; in Lim, Recent advances in otitis media with effusion: report of research conference. Ann. Otol. Rhinol. Lar. 94: suppl. 116, pp. 8–9 (1985).
10 Senturia, B.J.; Paparella, M.M.; Lowery, W.H.; et al.: Modified report of the ad hoc

committee on definition and classification of otitis media; in Lim, Report of research conference: recent advances in otitis media with effusion. Ann. Otol. Rhinol. Lar. *89:* suppl. 69, pp. 6–8 (1980).

11   Gates, G.A.; Paradise, J.L.; Birck, H.G.; et al.: Panel 7: Management; in Lim, Recent advances in otitis media with effusion: report of research conference. Ann. Otol. Rhinol. Lar. *94:* suppl. 116, pp. 27–30 (1985).

12   Tos, M.; Poulsen, G.: Screening tympanometry in infants and two-year-old children. Ann. Otol. Rhinol. Lar. *89:* suppl. 68, pp. 217–222 (1980).

13   Fiellau-Nikolajsen, M.: Tympanometry in three-year-old children: prevalence and spontaneous course of MEE. Ann. Otol. Rhinol. Lar. *89:* suppl. 68, pp. 223–227 (1980).

14   Lous, J.; Fiellau-Nikolajsen, M.: Epidemiology of middle-ear effusion and tubal dysfunction. A one-year prospective study comprising monthly tympanometry in 387 non-selected seven-year-old children. Int. J. pediat. Otorhinolar. *3:* 303–317 (1981).

15   Thomsen, J.; Tos, M.: Spontaneous improvement of secretory otitis: A long-term study. Acta oto-lar. *92:* 493–499 (1981).

16   Tos, M.; Melchiors, H.; Thomsen, J.; Plate, S.: Changes of the drum in untreated secretory otitis and chronic tubal dysfunction. Acta oto-lar., suppl. 386, pp. 149–151 (1982).

17   Thomsen, J.; Tos, M.; Hancke, A.B.; Melchiors, H.: Repetitive tympanometric screenings in children followed from birth to age four. Acta oto-lar., suppl. 386, pp. 155–157 (1982).

18   Tos, M.; Holm-Jensen, S.; Sørensen, C.H.; Mogensen, C.: Spontaneous course and frequency of secretory otitis in 4-year-old children. Archs Otolar. *108:* 4–10 (1982).

19   Fiellau-Nikolajsen, M.: Epidemiology of secretory otitis media. A descriptive cohort study. Ann. Otol. Rhinol. Lar. *92:* 172–177 (1983).

20   Tos, M.; Stangerup, S.-E.; Andreassen, U.K.; Hvid, G.; Thomsen, J.; Holm-Jensen, S.: Natural history of secretory otitis media; in Lim, Bluestone, Klein, Nelson, Recent advances in otitis media with effusion, pp. 36–40 (Decker, Philadelphia 1984).

21   Marchant, C.D.; Shurin, P.A.; Turczyk, V.A.; Wasikowski, D.E.; Tutihasi, M.A.; Kinney, S.E.: Course and outcome of otitis media in early infancy: a prospective study. J. Pediat. *104:* 826–831 (1984).

22   Bluestone, C.D.; Beery, Q.C.; Paradise, J.L.: Audiometry and tympanometry in relation to middle-ear effusions in children. Laryngoscope *83:* 594–604 (1972).

23   Fria, T.J.; Cantekin, E.I.; Eichler, J.A.: Hearing acuity of children with otitis media with effusion. Archs Otolar. *111:* 10–16 (1985).

24   Editorial: The glue-ear syndrome. Lancet *ii:* 397–398 (1975).

25   Paparella, M.M.; Oda, M.; Hiraide, F.; Brady, D.: Pathology of sensorineural hearing loss in otitis media. Ann. Otol. Rhinol. Lar. *81:* 632–647 (1972).

26   Paparella, M.M.; Goycoolea, M.V.; Meyerhoff, W.L.: Inner ear pathology and otitis media. A review. Ann. Otol. Rhinol. Lar. *89:* suppl. 68, pp. 249–253 (1972).

27   Paradise, J.L.: Otitis media during early life. How hazardous to development? A critical review of the evidence. Pediatrics, Springfield *68:* 869–873 (1981).

28   Hubbard, T.W.; Paradise, J.L.; McWilliams, B.J.; Elster, B.A.; Taylor, F.H.: Consequences of unremitting middle ear disease in early life: otologic, audiologic, and

developmental findings in children with cleft palate. New Engl. J. Med. *312:* 1529–1534 (1985).

29 Cantekin, E.I.; Mandel, E.M.; Bluestone, C.D.; Rockette, H.E.; Paradise, J.L.; Stool, S.E.; Fria, T.J.; Rogers, K.D.: Lack of efficacy of a decongestant-antihistamine combination for otitis media with effusion ('secretory' otitis media) in children. Results of a double-blind, randomized trial. New Engl. J. Med. *308:* 297–301 (1983).

30 Mandel, E.M.; Rockette, H.E.; Bluestone, C.D.; Paradise, J.L.; Nozza, R.J.: Efficacy of amoxicillin with and without decongenstant-antihistamine for otitis media with effusion in children. Results of a double-blind, randomized trial. New Engl. J. Med. *316:* 432–437 (1987).

31 Marks, M.J.; Mills, R.P.; Shaheen, O.H.: A controlled trial of contrimoxazole therapy in serous otitis media. J. Lar. Otol. *95:* 1003–1009 (1981).

32 Healy, G.B.: Antimicrobial therapy of chronic otitis media with effusion. Int. J. pediat. Otolar. *8:* 13–17 (1984).

33 Fraser, J.G.; Mehta, M.; Fraser, P.M.: The medical treatment of secretory otitis media. A clinical trial of three commonly used regimes. J. Lar. Otol. *91:* 757–765 (1977).

34 Grote, J.J.; Kuijpers, W.: Middle-ear effusion and sinusitis. J. Lar. Otol. *94:* 177–183 (1980).

35 Lildholdt, T.; Kortholm, B.: Beclomethasone nasal spray in the treatment of middle-ear effusion. A double-blind study. Int. J. pediat. Otorhinolar. *4:* 133–137 (1982).

36 Mawson, S.R.; Fagan, P.: Tympanic effusions in children: long-term results of treatment by myringotomy, aspiration and indwelling tubes (grommets). J. Lar. Otol. *86:* 105–119 (1972).

37 Kilby, D.; Richards, S.H.; Hart, G.: Grommets and glue ears. Two year results. J. Lar. Otol. *86:* 881–888 (1972).

38 Kokko, E.: Chronic secretory otitis media in children. Acta otolar., suppl. 327, pp. 7–44 (1974).

39 Hussl, B.; cited by Kokko, E.: Chronic secretory otitis media in children. Acta otolar., suppl 327, p. 7 (1974).

40 Cowan, D.L.; Brown, M.J.K.M.: Seromucinous otitis media and its sequelae (a retrospective study of 242 children). J. Lar. Otol. *88:* 1237–1247 (1974).

41 Tos, M.; Poulsen, G.: Secretory otitis media. Late results of treatment with grommets. Archs Otolar. *102:* 672–675 (1976).

42 Brown, M.J.K.M.; Richards, S.H.; Ambegaokar, A.G.: Grommets and glue ear. A five-year follow-up of a controlled trial. J. R. Soc. Med. *71:* 353–356 (1978).

43 Barfoed, C.; Rosborg, J.: Secretory otitis media. Long-term observations after treatment with grommets. Archs Otolar. *106:* 553–556 (1980).

44 Lildholdt, T.: Ventilation tubes in secretory otitis media. A randomized, controlled study of the course, the complications, and the sequelae of ventilation tubes. Acta oto-lar., suppl. 398, pp. 5–28 (1983).

45 Tos, M.; Bonding, P.; Poulsen, G.: Tympanosclerosis of the drum in secretory otitis after insertion of grommets. A prospective, comparative study. J. Lar. Otol. *97:* 489–496 (1983).

46 Bonding, P.; Tos, M.: Grommets versus paracentesis in secretory otitis media. A prospective, controlled study. Am. J. Otol. *6:* 455–460 (1985).

47 Tos, M.: Upon the relationship between secretory otitis in childhood and chronic otitis and its sequelae in adults. J. Lar. Otol. *95:* 1011–1022 (1981).

48 Richards, S.H.; Kilby, D.; Shaw, J.D.; et al.: Grommets and glue ears; a clinical trial.
    J. Lar. Otol. *85:* 17–22 (1971).
49 MacKinnon, D.M.: The sequel to myringotomy for exudative otitis media. J. Lar.
    Otol. *85:* 773–793 (1971).
50 Yagi, H.I.A.: The surgical treatment of secretory otitis media in children. J. Lar.
    Otol. *91:* 267–270 (1977).
51 Mandel, E.M.; Bluestone, C.D.; Paradise, J.L.; Cantekin, E.; Rockette, H.E.; Fria,
    T.J.; Stool, S.E.; Marshak, G.: Efficacy of myringotomy with and without tympanos-
    tomy tube insertion in the treatment of chronic otitis media with effusion in infants
    and children: results for the first year of a randomized clinical trial; in Lim, Blues-
    tone, Klein, Nelson, Recent advances in otitis media with effusion, pp. 308–312
    (Decker, Philadelphia 1984).
52 McKee, W.J.E.: A controlled study of the effects of tonsillectomy and adenoidec-
    tomy in children. Br. J. prev. soc. Med. *17:* 49–69 (1963).
53 McKee, W.J.E.: The part played by adenoidectomy in the combined operation of
    tonsillectomy with adenoidectomy. Second part of a controlled study in children. Br.
    J. prev. soc. Med. *17:* 133–140 (1963).
54 Mawson, S.R.; Adlington, P.; Evans, M.: A controlled study evaluation of adeno-
    tonsillectomy in children. J. Lar. Otol. *81:* 777–790 (1967).
55 Rynnel-Dagöö, B.; Ahlbom, A.; Schiratzki, H.: Effects of adenoidectomy. A con-
    trolled two-year follow-up. Ann. Otol. Rhinol. Lar. *87:* 272–278 (1978).
56 Roydhouse, N.: Adenoidectomy for otitis media with mucoid effusion. Ann. Otol.
    Rhinol. Lar. *89:* suppl. 68, pp. 312–315 (1980).
57 Feillau-Nikolajsen, M.; Hojslet, P.-E.; Felding, J.V.: Adenoidectomy for eustachian
    tube dysfunction: long-term results from a randomized controlled trial. Acta oto-lar.,
    suppl. 386, pp. 129–131 (1982).
58 Widemar, L.; Rynnel-Dagoo, B.; Schiratzki, H.; Svensson, C.: The effect of adenoid-
    ectomy on secretory otitis media. Acta oto-lar., suppl. 386, pp. 132–133 (1982).
59 Maw, A.R.: Chronic otitis media with effusion (glue ear) and adenotonsillectomy.
    Prospective randomized controlled study. Br. med. J. *287:* 1586–1588 (1983).
60 Bulman, C.H.; Brook, S.J.; Berry, M.G.: A prospective randomized trial of adenoid-
    ectomy vs. grommet insertion in the treatment of glue ear. Clin. Otolar. *9:* 67–75
    (1984).
61 Black, N.; Crowther, J.; Freeland, A.: The effectiveness of adenoidectomy in the
    treatment of glue ear. A randomized controlled trial. Clin. Otolar. *11:* 149–155
    (1986).
62 Maw, A.R.; Herod, F.: Otoscopic, impedance, and audiometric findings in glue ear
    treated by adenoidectomy and tonsillectomy. Lancet *i:* 1399–1402 (1986).
63 Paradise, J.L.; Bluestone, C.D.; Rogers, K.D.; Taylor, F.H.; Colborn, D.K.; Bach-
    man, R.Z.; Bernard, B.S.; Smith, C.G.; Stool, S.E.; Schwarzbach, R.H.: Efficacy of
    adenoidectomy for recurrent otitis media. Results from parallel random and non-
    random trials (Abstract). Pediat. Res. *21:* 286A (1987).

Jack L. Paradise, MD, Departments of Pediatrics and Community Medicine,
University of Pittsburgh School of Medicine, Children's Hospital of Pittsburgh,
One Children's Place, 3705 Fifth Avenue at DeSoto Street,
Pittsburgh, PA 15213 (USA)

Cholesteatoma

Adv. Oto-Rhino-Laryng., vol. 40, pp. 110–117 (Karger, Basel 1988)

Incidence, Etiology and Pathogenesis of Cholesteatoma in Children

M. Tos

ENT Department, Gentofte University Hospital, Hellerup, Denmark

The literature contains conflicting reports on the pathogenesis and classification of cholesteatomas in both children and adults [1]. There appears, however, to be universal agreement that cholesteatoma growth is more aggressive and rapid in children than in adults. Furthermore, in children cholesteatoma is often located in a non-sclerotic cell system, as opposed to adults. This study presents my clinical arguments in favor of the retraction theory [2] and in favor of the assumption that by far the majority of cholesteatomas, in children as well as adults, result from secretory otitis, which causes atrophy of the tympanic membrane and retraction pockets that at a later stage develop into cholesteatoma [3].

Definitions

To subdivide cholesteatomas into primary and secondary ones is, in my view, unsatisfactory because it presupposes a certain pathogenetic theory for the development of primary attic cholesteatomas and another for the development of secondary tensa cholesteatomas [4].

A subdivision of cholesteatomas into attic cholesteatomas, Shrapnell's membrane cholesteatomas and tensa cholesteatomas, respectively, according to their site of origin is in my view both logical and simple, being based exclusively on otoscopy [1]. I furthermore suggest a subdivision of tensa cholesteatomas into sinus cholesteatomas, i.e., those extending from the posterosuperior quadrant of pars tensa and spreading toward the stapes and tympanic sinus, and tensa retraction cholesteatomas [3], i.e., those originating from a retraction of the whole inferior part of the tympanic membrane [1].

Table I. Incidence (per year and per 100,000 population) of cholesteatoma

Cholesteatoma type	Children		Adults		Total	
	n	incidence year/ 100,000, %	n	incidence year/ 100,000, %	n	incidence year/ 100,000, %
Attic	49	1.0	224	4.7	273	5.7
Sinus	62	1.3	209	4.4	271	5.7
Tensa	26	0.5	170	3.5	196	4.1
Total	137	2.9	603	12.6	740	15.5

Relation children:adults, 1:5.
Number of cholesteatomas operated during the 16-year period from a population of 300,000 inhabitants.

Incidence

On the basis of 137 cholesteatomas in children aged 3–14 years and 603 cholesteatomas in adults (15–80 years), operated on during a period of 16 years from 1965 through 1980, in an area comprising 300,000 inhabitants, the annual incidence of cholesteatoma was calculated to be about 3 in children and 12.6 in adults per 100,000 inhabitants (table I).

Cholesteatomas in children account for 19% of the entire series and the ratio children:adults is thus 1:5. As the cholesteatomas in children were encountered over a period of 14 years (18%) and those in adults over a span of 66 years (82%) the mean annual incidence is the same for children and adults.

The incidence of the different types of cholesteatomas shows only minor variations in adults (table I), although the incidence of tensa retraction cholesteatoma is somewhat lower than that of the other two types. In children the incidence of tensa retraction cholesteatomas is about half that of attic cholesteatomas, and sinus cholesteatoma is the most frequently encountered type.

Ossicular chain pathology in children (table II) does not vary significantly from that found in adults. As expected, ossicular chain pathology is most pronounced in ears with tensa retraction cholesteatoma, and this applies to children as well as to adults.

Pathogenesis

The epidemiologic studies performed during recent years, in which cohorts of otherwise healthy children were followed from birth until school age and repeatedly examined with tympanometry and otomicroscopy, have enabled us to analyze the prevalence and severity of the various sequelae of the tympanic membrane (table III, IV) as well as to follow their possible progression [5].

Table II. Gross pathology of the ossicular chain in cholesteatoma in children, compared to adults

Cholesteatoma type	Intact %	Stapes present %	Stapes absent %
Attic (n = 49)	18	59	22
Sinus (n = 62)	15	55	31
Tensa (n = 26)	8	58	35
Children (n = 137)	15	57	28
Adults (n = 603)	18	49	33

Table III. Prevalence of attic retractions at different ages in a randomized cohort compared to two clinical materials of children with secretory otitis treated by grommets and adenoidectomy, and reevaluated 3–8 years and again 10–16 and 11–18 years after treatment

Type of retraction	Randomized cohort, age			Treated secretory otitis (years postop.)		
	5 years (n = 444) %	7 years (n = 444) %	10 years (n = 470) %	material I		material II
				3–8 years (n = 527), %	10–16 years (n = 362), %	11–18 years (n = 178), %
I	9.2	11.5	10.6	12.7	9.4	13.5
II	7.0	13.7	11.1	17.3	9.9	14.6
III	1.1	3.4	4.3	3.4	5.8	4.5
IV	0.7	0.9	0.4	0.8	1.7	1.7
Attic cholesteatoma	–	–	–	0.2	0.6	1.7
Total	18.0	29.5	26.4	34.4	27.4	36.0
χ^2 test	$p < 0.05$	n.s.		$p < 0.01$	$p < 0.05$	

Patients treated for secretory otitis by insertion of ventilation tubes and adenotomy during the years 1970–1974 have been reexamined twice, first 3–8 years after surgery [6, 7], and again 10–16 years after treatment (material I) [8]. In another series (material II), patients were treated in the same way during the period from 1965 to 1970 and reexamined 11–18 years postoperatively [9]. A comparison of the prevalence of tympanic membrane pathology renders it possible to make a clinical evaluation of the validity of the various pathogenetic theories.

Attic Cholesteatoma and Attic Retraction

Attic cholesteatomas extend from the region of Shrapnell's membrane and are always primarily located in the attic [10, 11]. All series showed a high prevalence of attic retractions, which were divided into types I–IV. In a few ears attic cholesteatoma was already present, which was verified at operation (table III). Type I indicates a harmless retraction of Shrapnell's membrane, and type II a retraction extending to the malleus head. In type III there is some resorption of the bony annulus and the retracted Shrapnell's membrane appears larger than normal. A

Table IV. Prevalence of changes of pars tensa at different ages in a randomized cohort compared to two clinical materials of children with secretory otitis, treated by grommets and adenoidectomy, and reevaluated 3–8 years after and again 10–16 years and 11–18 years after treatment

Type of pathology	Randomized cohort, age			Treated secretory otitis (years postop.)		
	5 years (n = 444) %	7 years (n = 444) %	10 years (n = 470) %	material I		material II
				3–8 years (n = 527), %	10–16 years (n = 362), %	11–18 years (n = 178), %
Atrophy	2.5	6.3	8.1	21.3	11.4	14.6
Atrophy and pexy	0.7	2.0	2.3	3.2	4.7	10.1
Adhesive otitis	–	–	–	2.5	2.2	3.9
Sinus cholesteatoma	–	–	–	–	0.3	–
Atrophy with perforation	0.2	0.2	0.2	–	–	1.7
Atrophy with tympanosclerosis	0.7	1.4	2.3	9.1	10.8	9.6
Tympanosclerosis only	4.7	7.2	5.1	18.8	25.7	18.5
Abnormal pars tensa	8.8	17.1	18.0	54.8	58.1	58.4
χ^2 test	p < 0.001		p < 0.001		n.s.	

type-IV retraction indicates pronounced resorption of bone and Shrapnell's membrane is retracted down onto the malleus head. Most of the retractions were harmless, but severe retractions were encountered in 4% of the 10-year-old, otherwise healthy children (table III) and in 8% of the patients in material II. Thus, the incidence of severe attic retractions in children is several times higher than that of attic cholesteatoma (table I, III) and the risk of further progression into cholesteatoma is present. Peroperatively, it is often quite evident that the attic cholesteatoma is in fact a retraction of Shrapnell's membrane. The development of an attic cholesteatoma from an attic retraction might conceivably be initiated by impairment of the transport route from the retraction caused by some banal hindrance such as cerumen or external otitis. This results in accumulation of debris in the retraction, infection and crust formation, which eventually closes the retraction and further promotes the infection. In this precholesteatomatous condition, proliferation of cells in the germinative layer appears to be a logical explanation of the progression of the retraction and growth of the cholesteatoma. In this way, the retraction theory [2] can be combined with the proliferation theory [12]. In my view, however, both retraction and infection of the retraction pocket are prerequisites of proliferation of the cells in Shrapnell's membrane [10]. The retraction theory is supported by the fact that recurrent cholesteatoma develops after combined approach tympanoplasty which always starts as a retraction.

With regard to attic cholesteatoma, the immigration theory [4], which presupposes a marginal perforation, completely lacks clinical documentation. In our three cohorts we have never encountered a perforation of Shrapnell's membrane in association with acute otitis.

Sinus Cholesteatoma and Posterosuperior Retraction

Sinus cholesteatoma is in fact a primary tensa cholesteatoma originating in a posterosuperior retraction which extends down onto the incudostapedial joint, the stapes, and into the tympanic sinus. From here, it spreads medially to the incudal body and the malleus head up toward the attic and aditus [3, 10]. In 26% of the children the sinus cholesteatoma was confined to the tympanic cavity; in 29% it extended to the aditus and the attic; in 34% also to antrum, and in 11% to the mastoid process. In clinical series of children we have often observed the following development of sinus cholesteatoma from a posterosuperior retraction: impaired migration from a posterosuperior retraction causes accumulation of debris in the retraction and infection. The formation of a crust seals off the retraction and promotes the infection of the retraction. The keratinized squamous epithelium proliferates, debris continues to accumulate and the retraction increases in size. Although atrophy and retraction, especially in children, are caused by a long-standing negative middle ear pressure [16], spread of the retraction may occur in ears with a normal middle ear pressure and normal tubal function.

In randomized cohorts of children, atrophy was found in 3% of 5-year-old children increasing to 10% in children aged 10; 2% of the ears in addition had posterior atrophy with retraction as well as pexy to the stapes (table IV). In a clinical series of patients with secretory otitis, eardrum pathology was found in more than half of the ears and atrophy in about 30%. In the oldest series, posterior atrophy and pexy were found in 10% of the ears and adhesive otitis in 4%. In these ears there is a constant risk of later progression and development of primary sinus cholesteatoma or primary tensa retraction cholesteatoma.

Tensa Retraction Cholesteatoma

This group represents patients in whom the entire tympanic membrane was primarily adherent to the medial wall of the tympanic cavity [3, 10].

In typical cases, the cholesteatoma membrane lines the whole tympanic cavity and the tubal orifice, and invests the malleus handle which is often resorbed [11]. The cholesteatoma spreads medially to the incus and malleus up towards the attic and aditus. In my view, the retraction theory fully explains the development of tensa cholesteatoma [1]. Diffuse atrophy and retraction of the whole eardrum (atelectasis) is a well-known sequela to secretory otitis. Pars tensa is flaccid, too big and adherent to the medial wall of the tympanic cavity. At the same time, there is often myringostapediopexy (table IV). Tubal occlusion may lead to further retraction and if infection intervenes, the membrane may become adherent. The impaired self-cleaning mechanism of the retraction causes accumulation of debris and crust formation in the tympanic cavity. In this precholesteatomatous condition, the retractions spread up towards the attic and the end result is, irreversibly, cholesteatoma. This development of tensa retraction cholesteatoma may be observed clinically, and at surgery it is often quite evident that the original condition was a retraction rather than a perforation.

Discussion and Conclusion

Among 191 patients with cleft palates, who were followed for many years, the incidence of cholesteatoma was 9.2%, the main reason for which, it is universally agreed, is poor tubal function [14]. A study from Iowa [15] showed annual incidences of 6 cholesteatomas/100,000 inhabitants, which is considerably lower than the incidence found in the present study (table I). To my knowledge, the literature contains no reference to the incidence of cholesteatoma among children, but among high-risk populations in Queensland, Australia, the incidence of cholesteatomas was 0.1% [16].

In our series of patients with secretory otitis, followed up over several years, there was a high prevalence of eardrum pathology, especially atrophy, which may later progress. Improvement of the tubal function following abatement of secretory otitis does not in itself ensure improvement of atrophy, pexy or adhesions. Thus, the risk of later progression persists.

The immigration theory [4], or the marginal perforation theory, has not been substantiated by our epidemiologic or clinical studies. According to this theory, acute otitis – especially in association with measles and scarlatina – should give rise to necrosis of the tympanic membrane and a marginal perforation, permitting in the course of restoration the epithelium of the outer ear canal to grow into the tympanic membrane. Our epidemiological studies show that 90% of all children have at least one episode of acute otitis, but all perforations closed spontaneously, as demonstrated by follow-up tympanometry and otomicroscopy. Children's diseases do not in the Western world give rise to eardrum perforations, and especially not peripheral perforations. The acute peripheral perforation is in my opinion a myth; at least we have never encountered one, either in Shrapnell's membrane or in pars tensa.

There can be no major pathogenetic differences between children and adults; in children, however, the mastoid process is better pneumatized and sclerosis is rarer than in adults [17]. The explanation for this may be that the sclerotic process forms part of the cholesteatomatous disease process, which in adults has been of considerably longer duration than in children.

References

1   Schwarz, M.: Cholesteatom im Gehörgang und im Mittelohr, pp. 1–187 (Thieme, Stuttgart 1966).

2   Bezold, F.: Über das Cholesteatom des Mittelohrs. Z. Ohrenheilk. *21:* 252–263 (1891).

3   Tos, M.: Relationship between secretory otitis in childhood and chronic otitis and its sequelae in adults. J. Lar. Otol. *95:* 1011–1022 (1981).

4   Habermann, J.: Zur Entstehung des Cholesteatoms des Mittelohres. Arch. Ohrenheilk. *27:* 42–56 (1889).

5   Tos, M.; Hvid, G.; Stangerup, S.-E.; Andreassen, U.K.: Prevalence and progressions of sequelae after secretory otitis. Ann. Otol. Rhinol. Lar. (in press, 1988).

6   Tos, M.; Poulsen, G.: Attic retractions following secretory otitis. Acta oto-lar. *89:* 479–486 (1980).

7   Tos, M.; Poulsen, G.: Changes of pars tensa after secretory otitis. ORL *41:* 313–328 (1979).

8   Tos, M.; Stangerup, S.-E.; Larsen, P.: Dynamics of attic retractions and changes of pars tensa following secretory otitis. A prospective study. Archs Otolar. *113:* 380–385 (1987).

9   Tos, M.; Larsen, P.; Siim, C.: Trommehindeforandringer efter sekretorisk otitis og deres relation til kronisk otitis. Ugeskr. Læg. (in press, 1988).

10 Tos, M.: Can cholesteatoma be prevented? in Sadé, Cholesteatoma and mastoid surgery, pp. 591–597 (Kugler, Amsterdam 1982).

11 Tos, M.: Pathology of the ossicular chain in various chronic middle ear diseases. J. Otol. Rhinol. Lar. *93:* 769–780 (1979).

12 Rüedi, L.: Cholesteatosis of the attic. J. Otolar. *72:* 593–609 (1958).

13 Tos, M.; Stangerup, S.-E.; Holm-Jensen, S.; Sørensen, C.H.: Spontaneous course of secretory otitis and changes of the eardrum. Archs Otolar. *110:* 281–289 (1984).

14 Harker, L.A.; Severeid, L.R.: Cholesteatoma in the cleft palate patients; in Sadé, Cholesteatoma and mastoid surgery, pp. 37–40 (Kugler, Amsterdam 1977).

15 Harker, L.A.: Cholesteatoma: an incidence study; in McCabe, Sadé, Abramson, Cholesteatoma: First International Conference, pp. 308–312 (1977).

16 McCafferty, G.J.; Coman, W.B.; Shaw, E.; Lewis, N.: Cholesteatoma in Australian Aboriginal children; in McCabe, Sadé, Abramson, Cholesteatoma: First International Conference, pp. 293–301 (1977).

17 Rüedi, L.: Pathogenesis and treatment of cholesteatoma in chronic suppuration of the temporal bone. Ann. Otol. Rhinol. Lar. *66:* 285 (1957).

M. Tos, MD, ENT Department, Gentofte University Hospital,
DK–2900 Hellerup (Denmark)

Adv. Oto-Rhino-Laryng., vol. 40, pp. 118–123 (Karger, Basel 1988)

Retraction Pocket and Development of Cholesteatoma in Children

C.R. Pfaltz

Department of ORL, University Hospital of Basel, Basel, Switzerland

According to Schuknecht [1974] a retraction pocket consists of an invagination of a replacement membrane into the middle ear space and may occur either in the pars tensa or Shrapnell's membrane. A retraction pocket may be 'fixed', i.e. adherent to the structures in the middle ear, or 'mobile', i.e. free to move in response to pressure differences acting upon the membrane. A retraction pocket may sometimes also be a *potential* or *prospective cholesteatoma* but the crucial diagnostic problem arises if we have to answer the question: When does a retraction pocket become a cholesteatoma?

According to Sadé [1982] some retraction pockets are either simple and shallow and often self-cleansing, whereas others may accumulate keratin and are infected. He does not consider them already real cholesteatomas and advises to treat them by suction cleaning. Or the retraction pocket is deep, not self cleansing, infected for a long time, extending into the antrum or the oval window region and very often causing a partial destruction of the incus. They are considered true cholesteatomas and therefore surgery is advised. Nager [1977] distinguishes a *postero-superior tensa retraction pocket* from a *central form of location.* In our material the latter form is rather unfrequent and shall not be discussed further. The postero-superior tensa retraction pocket, however, is very frequently observed, both in children and in adults. Its relation to adjacent bony structures predisposes to a development into and enlargement within the tympanic cavity.

Pathogenetic Aspects

Chronic impairment of middle ear ventilation causes reversible retraction of the pars tensa but intermittent middle ear infections lead to atrophy and further retraction *(potential cholesteatoma)*; if it becomes irreversible due to adherence to the promontory or the long crus of the incus it is considered a *prospective cholesteatoma*. Every time a virulent infection is spread from the upper respiratory tract to the middle ear cavity the mucoperiosteum is inflamed, becomes hyperplastic and impairs middle ear ventilation additionally. If this inflammation of the tympanic mucosa becomes chronic and the retraction pocket irreversible the mucosa will then be gradually transformed into a *perimatrix* by losing its epithelial covering. It will get into close contact and finally becomes adherent to the atrophic membrane of the deep tensa pocket, which then becomes the *matrix* of the *tensa cholesteatoma*. Because a deep irreversible, fixed retraction pocket has lost its natural self-cleansing mechanism (successful outward migration), keratin is collected in this pocket and this debris becomes infected, particularly by gram-negative proteolytic bacteria (proteus or pyocyaneus). Their endotoxins are activating papillary growth of the squamous epithelium within the retraction pocket, which has become the *matrix* of the *active tensa cholesteatoma*. At the same time they activate the precursor cells of osteoclasts within the *perimatrix,* initiating the bone resorption or osteolytic process characteristic of the active cholesteatoma. The question is still open why some of the retraction pockets remain potential cholesteatomas, i.e. inactive, and why others become prospective and finally active tensa cholesteatomas? Three factors seem to play a prevalent part in the pathogenesis of tensa cholesteatoma.

(1) Disturbance of Middle Ear Ventilation and Drainage

Bluestone et al. [1982] concluded from the results of their study in 27 children that all of the subjects with an acquired cholesteatoma or a retraction pocket, regardless of site, had functional obstruction of the Eustachian tube. These authors emphasize that a retraction pocket, either in the postero-superior quadrant or of the pars flaccida, should be considered a precursor of acquired cholesteatoma. In their opininon this makes aggressive management of such retraction pockets important in prevention of this disease.

Buckingham [1982] does not agree with this statement. He considers deep retraction pockets, forced into the middle ear by atmospheric pressure greater than middle ear pressure, reversible *pulsion diverticula* of atrophic areas of pars tensa. According to his observations middle ear ventilation and local therapy permit these pulsion diverticula to recede, shrink and return to the annular plane. According to our own findings, based on a long-term follow-up study [Hug and Pfaltz, 1980], we cannot confirm this view. In this previous study, based on an average follow-up period of > 2 years in 25 children (50 ears) suffering from recurrent otitis media with effusion, we were able to demonstrate: 31 normal tympanic membranes; 15 atrophic parts of the pars tensa (post. sup. quadrant); 2 deep retraction pockets; 1 marginal perforation, and 1 tensa cholesteatoma.

All these children had been treated over a longer period of time by repeated insertion of a grommet. The tensa cholesteatoma developed gradually within a period of 5 years and had to be operated. We therefore support firmly Bluestone's strategy of aggressive management of deep irreversible and fixed retraction pockets. The failure of middle ear drainage and ventilation may be explained by the fact that meso- and hypotympanum can be easily ventilated, the narrow compartments of the epitympanic space and the antrum cannot be aerated because they are filled with a hyperplastic mucosa and retained secretions. An inflammatory process will persist in this part of the middle ear and contribute to further impairment of ventilation, i.e. a vicious circle will develop, resulting in atrophic scars of the pars tensa, retraction pockets and finally in a tensa cholesteatoma.

(2) Disturbance of Epithelial Migration in Retraction Pockets

Makino and Amatsu [1986] made the following observation experimentally and clinically: When blood supply of the pars tensa and the external canal is poor, the epidermal metabolism will be lowered and as a result disturb epithelial migration. They found that less-vascularized tympanic membranes with atrophy or calcification showed slowing of the epithelial migratory rate, abnormal migratory patterns and desquamation. These findings indicate that a poor blood supply is the major etiologic factor for the migratory disturbance in retraction pockets, resulting in a loss of its natural self-cleansing mechanism.

(3) Destruction of the Fibrous and Osseous Tympanic Annulus

The tympanic membrane is fixed in a circular groove of the tympanic bone (tympanic sulcus of the annulus tympanicus osseus) by the fibrous annulus. The latter consists of several circular layers of collagene fibre bundles. It is missing in the area of Rivini's notch. This is the only part of the tympanic membrane where the epidermis of the external canal turns directly into the epidermal layer of the drum without a shrarp demarcation line and where the drum is not tightened by the fibrous ring (pars flaccida) [Beck, 1979]. As long as the fibrous ring is intact failure of middle ear ventilation will only result in reversible retraction pockets, even if the membrane becomes atrophic. However, as soon as the fibrous annulus is destroyed by trauma or inflammation the adjacent part of the pars tensa is no longer tightened and will be retracted permanently in case of intratympanic hypoventilation. Moreover, keratin debris accumulation, an ideal culture medium for microorganisms, will induce stimulation of papillary growth of meatal epidermis by endotoxins. Because the collagen fibre bundle barrier is missing thus allowing unimpeded papillary downgrowth of keratinizing squamous epithelium into the middle ear, the development of tensa cholesteatoma with a typical marginal perforation in the posterosuperior quadrant is initiated.

Therapeutic Aspects

In the current literature there is little agreement whether a retraction pocket should be operated at all or only healed by long-term ventilation of the middle ear. Eliachar and Joachims [1982] emphasize that localized atelectatic retraction pockets signal the alarm of impending irreversible complications. Re-establishment of adequate middle ear ventilation is from the view of these authors the key in every attempt to arrest and reverse this pathology. They present the result of a study on 177 advanced cases in which they were able to demonstrate the reversibility of a seemingly irreversible pathology in the middle ear, achieved by the application of long term silicon ventilating tubes.

In our opinion this type of management should always be tried in *children,* before a more invasive type of ear surgery is performed. In *adults,* however, I should like to enumerate the following indications for tympanoplasty: (1) impaired self-cleansing mechanism of the retraction pocket (intermittent discharge); (2) granulation at the posterosuperior margin of the tympanic annulus and apparent destruction of the fibrous annulus; (3) considerable conductive hearing loss; (4) the pocket is formed by an atrophic membrane, floating back and forth with respiration, thus causing annoying noises or even painful sensations.

Portmann [1982] has based his indications for surgical treatment of retraction pockets on the following criteria: Anatomical structure of the mastoid (reduced pneumatization), functional state, extension of the local lesion and the general condition of the patient. He summarizes that there is no method of choice for the management of retraction pockets and that the selection of a particular surgical technique for each particular case will always be a compromise. Sadé [1982] emphasizes that it is often not easy to distinguish between a large retraction pocket with an intact self-cleansing mechanism and an active tensa cholesteatoma originating from a deep pocket. He recommends to treat shallow retraction pockets with conservative methods (regular microscopic control with suction of the debris). Deep retraction pockets are removed by an endaural or retroauricular approach, if necessary with eradication of an infected 'dead space' in the region of the sinus tympani. His follow-up study or 308 atelectatic ears with retraction pockets showed that most of them did not progress but some of them even regressed. These findings account for the favorable prognosis of the conservatively treated and conservatively operated retraction pockets.

According to our own experience (long-term follow-up of more than 6 years) radical removal of a retraction pocket and reconstruction of the tympanic membrane demands the use of solid, resistant autologous grafting material, particularly in cases presenting a partially destroyed annulus tympanicus osseus and fibrosus. Both fascia and perichondrium do not have a structure which allows them to resist the retraction forces arising again postoperatively. Within a rather short time first a shallow and later a deep retraction pocket will form. We know from experience that autologous grafts like perichondrium and fascia are still the best material to be used for the reconstruction of the tympanic membrane, because they are biologically resistant and the take rate is high. If we need grafting material with more solid physical properties resisting retraction pocket repair, we use thin cartilage foils (taken from the tragus) which reinforce the tympanic graft without impairing its vibration properties [Pfaltz et al., 1982].

Conclusions

As soon as an atrophic part of the pars tensa becomes a retraction pocket, showing a tendency to accumulate keratin and debris and signs of repeated inflammation, it should be considered no longer a *potential* but a *prospective cholesteatoma* which will sooner or later turn into an *active tensa cholesteatoma*. In adults it should be operated before the patient's hearing is impaired by necrosis of the long process of the incus or parts of the stapes suprastructure. In children long time middle ear ventilation by insertion of a grommet should be tried first and surgical management (tympanoplasty with reinforcement of the marginal parts of the pars tensa) carried out only in cases of a fixed retraction pocket.

References

Beck, C.: Anatomie and Histologie des Ohres; in Berendes, Link, Zöllner, Hals-Nasen-Ohrenheilkunde in Praxis und Klinik, 2. Aufl., vol. V, Ohr, pp. 1–21 (Thieme, Stuttgart 1979).

Bluestone, C.D.; Chasselbrant, M.; Cantekin, E.I.: Functional obstruction of the Eustachian tube in the pathogenesis of aural cholesteatoma in children; in Sadé, Cholesteatoma and mastoid surgery, pp. 211–224 (Amsterdam 1982).

Buckingham, R.A.: The clinical appearance and natural history of cholesteatoma; in Sadé, Cholesteatoma and mastoid surgery, pp. 13–21 (Amsterdam 1982).

Eliachar, I.; Joachims, H.Z.: Arrest of cholesteatoma formation by long-term ventilation of the middle ear; in Sadé, Cholesteatoma and mastoid surgery, pp. 605–610 (Amsterdam 1982).

Hug, J.E.; Pfaltz, C.R.: Paukendrainage und Cholesteatom-Genese; in Aktuelle Probleme der Otorhinolaryngologie, vol. 3, pp. 9–15 (Huber, Bern 1980).

Makino, K.; Amatsu, M.: Epithelial migration on the tympanic membrane and external canal. German Archs Otorhinolar. *243:* 39–42 (1986).

Nager, G.D.: Cholesteatoma of the middle ear: pathogenesis and surgical indications; in McGabe, Sadé, Abramson, Cholesteatoma, 1st Int. Conf., Birmingham 1977, pp. 193–203.

Pfaltz, C.R.; Pfaltz, R.; Finkenzeller, P.: Short- and long-term results in ossiculo-plasty in cholesteatomatous ears; in Sadé, Cholesteatoma and mastoid surgery, pp. 559–566 (Amsterdam 1982).

Portmann, M.: Surgery of retraction pockets V.S. attic cholesteatoma. Is there a treatment of choice? in Sadé, Cholesteatoma and mastoid surgery, pp. 509–510 (Amsterdam 1982).

Sadé, J.: Treatment of retraction pockets and cholesteatoma; in Cholesteatoma and mastoid surgery, pp. 511–525 (Amsterdam 1982).

Schuknecht, H.F.: Pathology of the ear, pp. 218–220 (Harvard University Press, Cambridge 1974).

Prof. Dr. C.R. Pfaltz, Department of ORL, University Hospital of Basel, CH–4031 Basel (Switzerland)

Adv. Oto-Rhino-Laryng., vol. 40, pp. 124–130 (Karger, Basel 1988)

Surgery for Congenital and Acquired Cholesteatoma in Children

Mario Sanna, Carlo Zini, Roberto Gamoletti, Alessandra Russo, Roberta Scandellari, Abdel Taibah

Clinica Otorinolaringoiatrica 2°, Università di Parma, Parma, Italia

Introduction

The surgical approach to childhood cholesteatoma is still a controversial subject among otologists. Different approaches have been suggested by proponents of the canal-down technique [Baron, 1969; Charanchon et al., 1971; Palva et al., 1977; Abramson, 1985] and the canal-up technique [Armstrong, 1965; Goodey and Smyth, 1970; Sanna et al., 1976; Sheehy, 1978; Jansen, 1978; Smyth and Hassard, 1980; Zini and Sanna, 1980; Glasscock et al., 1981; Tos, 1983; Sanna et al., 1987], and they reflect the controversy in the treatment of adult acquired cholesteatoma.

Acquired cholesteatoma in children is the same disease that we find in adults. Congenital cholesteatoma on the contrary is a different entity which occurs much more frequently in children and has a different origin.

Classification of Cholesteatoma

Many classifications have been proposed in the literature but the etiopathogenetic distinction into acquired and congenital cholesteatoma remains valid.

Acquired cholesteatoma (secondary and primary) develops as a result of various factors such as otitis, trauma, tubal insufficiency and so on. Different theories have been proposed to explain the pathogenesis of this type of cholesteatoma including the theory of migration as a result of a marginal perforation of the eardrum, retraction of the tympanic membrane, proliferation of the germinative layer of Shrapnell's membrane and the theory of metaplasia of the mucous membrane.

Congenital cholesteatoma presumably results from embryonic inclusions of the squamous epithelium during the development of the temporal bone. This theory was first proposed by Korner in 1830. In accordance with Derlacki [1973], we use the term congenital to describe a cholesteatoma that develops inside the endotympanum and affects subjects whose histories record no event capable of favoring the migration of epidermal cells into the tympanic cavity. Congenital cholesteatoma must therefore be present behind a perfectly normal tympanic membrane in an ear showing no trace of prior inflammatory processes. For surgical management purposes we have differentiated three types of cholesteatomas according to the location: type A involving the mesotympanum; type B involving the epitympanum, and type AB mixed [Sanna and Zini, 1984].

Diagnosis

While the diagnosis of acquired cholesteatoma is generally easily made on inspection and rarely needs confirmation by X-ray studies, the detection of congenital middle ear cholesteatoma should start by suspecting it in children with unilateral conductive hearing impairment higher than 30–40 dB although their tympanic membrane is normal. The failure of medical treatment or of any transtympanic tube makes it necessary to perform an explorative tympanotomy. When patients complain of conductive hearing loss with no history of prior otitis, and a normal tympanic membrane and a whitish spot is found behind the drum, then congenital cholesteatoma is almost certainly present. For an early diagnosis of this condition, screening should be carried out in schools. Accurate testing of unilateral conductive hearing impairments in children enables the diagnosis of congenital cholesteatoma when it is still localized inside the tympanic cavity so as to prevent perforation of the tympanic membrane at a later stage which would add to complications during treatment.

Case Material

We have reviewed our series of 207 cases of childhood cholesteatoma operated on at our institution between January 1971 and December 1986. The series includes two groups of patients: 24 so-called congenital cholesteatomas (i.e. the presence of cholesteatoma behind a normal tympanic membrane in patients with no history of ear disease) and 183

Table I. Surgical techniques (207 cases)

	Number of cases	Staged ICWT	Non-staged ICWT	Open TPL	Radical mastoid-ectomy
Acquired cholesteatoma	183	147	24	4	8
Congenital cholesteatoma	24	19	5	–	–
Total	207	166	29	4	8

ICWT = Intact canal wall tympanoplasty; TPL = tympanoplasty.

acquired cholesteatomas (primary and secondary acquired) including 11 bilateral cases. The ages of the children considered herein ranged from 2.5 to 14 years.

A staged intact canal wall tympanoplasty (ICWT) was performed in 166 cases; a non-staged ICWT was done in 29 cases, and a radical mastoidectomy in 12 cases (4 modified plus 8 classic radical; table I). Acquired cholesteatomas included 43 type A, 44 type B, 88 type AB and 7 epidermizations. Congenital cholesteatomas included 12 type A and 12 type AB.

The present study is based on 178 cases with a minimum follow-up of 1 year (including 137 cases with a follow-up from 2 to 10 years).

Results

The results of cholesteatoma surgery are anatomical and curative as well as functional in terms of postoperative hearing results. Perforation of the tympanic graft occurred in 16 of 178 cases (9.0%), stenosis of the ear canal in 3 cases (1.7%) and atrophy of the posterior canal wall in 19 of 134 ICWT cases (14.2%).

The occurrence of residual cholesteatoma was only evaluated in the staged operations in which the second-look procedure was performed about 12 months after the first operation: this procedure is the only one to evaluate the real incidence of residual disease. One hundred and fifteen staged ICWTs and 4 open tympanoplasties were surgically reexplored in acquired cholesteatoma cases: 41 residual cholesteatomas were detected among 115 ICWTs (35.6%) and 2 residual cholesteatomas occurred among 4 open tympanoplasties (50%). The series of congenital cholesteatoma cases included 19 reexplored ICWTs and residual disease occurred in 10 cases (52.6%); in 1 case revision surgery was performed and again residual cholesteatoma was found totalling 11 out of 19 cases (57.9%; table II).

Table II. Residual cholesteatoma

	Reexplored cases	ICWT	Open TPL
Acquired cholesteatoma	119	41 of 115 (35.6%)	2 of 4 (50%)
Congenital cholesteatoma	19	10 of 19 (52.6%)	–
Total	138	51 of 134 (38.1%)	2 of 4 (50%)

ICWT = Intact canal wall tympanoplasty; TPL = tympanoplasty.

Table III. Recurrent cholesteatoma

	1-year follow-up			2- to 10-year follow-up		
	number of cases	ICWT	open TPL	number of cases	ICWT	open TPL
Acquired cholesteatoma	144	8 of 140 (5.7%)	1 of 4 (25%)	120	8 of 116 (6.9%)	1 of 4 (25%)
Congenital cholesteatoma	22	1[a] of 22 (4.5%)	–	17	3[a] of 17 (17.6%)	–
Total	166	9 of 162 (5.6%)	1 of 4 (25%)	137	11 of 133 (8.3%)	–

ICWT = Intact canal wall tympanoplasty; TPL = tympanoplasty.
[a] 1 case has been operated 3 times.

Recurrent cholesteatoma was detected in 9 of 144 acquired cholesteatomas with a follow-up of 1 year: 8 occurred among 140 ICWTs (5.7%) and 1 among the 4 open tympanoplasties (25%). At 2–10 years follow-up the incidence of recurrent cholesteatoma was 8 of 116 (6.9%) and 1 of 4 (25%) cases, respectively.

One case of recurrent cholesteatoma was detected in the series of 22 congenital cholesteatomas at 1 year follow-up (4.5%). At 2–10 years follow-up the incidence of recurrent cholesteatoma was 3 of 17 cases (17.6%; table III).

Post-operative hearing results in the series of both acquired and congenital cholesteatomas are reported in tables IV and V.

Table IV. Acquired cholesteatoma: functional results (100 cases)

	15 months	18 months	24 months	36 months	>48 months
0–15 dB	66 (66.0%)	51 (75.0%)	40 (71.4%)	20 (62.6%)	18 (69.3%)
16–25 dB	17 (17.0%)	9 (13.2%)	7 (12.5%)	6 (18.7%)	1 (3.8%)
>25 dB	17 (17.0%)	8 (11.8%)	9 (16.1%)	6 (18.7%)	7 (26.9%)

Table V. Congenital cholesteatoma: functional results (21 cases)

	15 months	18 months	24 months	36 months	>48 months
0–15 dB	12 (57.1%)	16 (76.2%)	12 (66.7%)	8 (53.4%)	6 (40.0%)
16–25 dB	6 (28.6%)	1 (4.8%)	2 (11.1%)	2 (13.3%)	2 (13.3%)
>25 dB	3 (14.3%)	4 (19.0%)	4 (22.2%)	5 (33.3%)	7 (46.7%)

Discussion

We consider acquired cholesteatoma in children as the same disease found in adults. Only the fact that it occurs in a different environment and is discovered and treated earlier justifies some differences in the clinical presentation of the disease.

Congenital cholesteatoma on the contrary is a completely different entity: the pathogenesis, the clinical presentation and presumably the natural course of the disease differ to a great extent when compared with the acquired counterpart. However, examination of our series, presented herein, shows some common aspects.

For both types of cholesteatoma there is no particular age for performing surgery in children: while a minimum age for operation can be accepted, there is no evidence that surgery should be deferred in children.

The presence of a large pneumatized mastoid in the child's ear has been considered by other surgeons as a situation conditioning the outcome of surgery and the type of surgery itself. We believe that ICWT is preferable in this instance because a normally healed ear can be obtained and minimal postoperative care is required.

The controversy on the treatment of choice for cholesteatoma in children continues and reflects the debate that is still raised by the treatment of cholesteatoma in adults: proponents of the open and closed techniques have all reported and discussed their results extensively.

We consider ICWT as the procedure of choice for childhood cholesteatoma both of the acquired and congenital type and it is a pre-planned staged procedure in 80% of cases in both instances. The possibility of preserving a nearly normal bony structure with the ICWT is particularly useful in congenital cholesteatoma cases in which it is often possible to preserve the patient's tympanic membrane. Congenital cholesteatoma in fact, especially in the early stages of its development, presents as a well-delineated cyst that can easily be dissected from the middle ear lining. However, the incidence of residual cholesteatoma appears to be increased among the congenital cholesteatoma cases because it is often deep-seated in the posterior mesotympanum. This is somewhat in contrast with the easy removal of congenital cholesteatoma from the middle ear cleft especially in the early stages of its development. We are still convinced that the identification and elimination of residual disease during preplanned second-stage procedures is not a complication or a failure but an inherent consequence of the canal-up philosophy. Recurrent cholesteatoma is increased on long-term follow-up among congenital cholesteatoma cases when compared with acquired cases, but we have no explanation for this finding. Our surgical technique has evolved towards the prevention of recurrent cholesteatoma with the use of Silastic sheeting and the repair of the posterior canal wall defects with cartilage shavings.

In conclusion we consider ICWT the procedure of choice for the treatment of childhood cholesteatoma. In our opinion staging of the operation is mandatory for detection and elimination of residual cholesteatoma which occurs more frequently in children than in adults [Sanna et al., 1987]. Meticulous attention should also be paid to correct all the situations that could otherwise lead to the formation of recurrent disease.

Congenital cholesteatoma appears less invasive in its early stages when compared with the acquired counterpart: this means preservation of the tympanic membrane in a greater number of cases. Anatomical results in terms of reperforations of the tympanic membrane, external ear canal stenosis and so on are thus better. The different characteristics of congenital cholesteatoma require an early diagnosis through extensive evaluation of all unilateral conductive hearing impairments greater than 30–40 dB occurring in children especially behind an intact tympanic membrane. It is our opinion that the incidence of congenital cholesteatoma is greater than reported.

We shall continue to use the staged ICWT because the end result is an essentially normal ear with good curative and functional results in 80% of our cases.

References

Abramson, M.: Open or closed tympanomastoidectomy for cholesteatoma in children. Am. J. Otol. *6:* 167–169 (1985).

Armstrong, B.W.: Tympanoplasty in children. Laryngoscope, St Louis *75:* 1062–1069 (1965).

Baron, S.H.: Management of aural cholesteatoma in children. Otolaryngol. Clin. North Am. *2:* 71–88 (1969).

Charanchon, R.; Junien-Lavillauroy, C.; Accoyer, B.: Indications de la tympanoplastie chez l'enfant. 68e Congr. fr. ORL, C.R., pp. 155–168 (1971).

Derlacki, E.L.: Congenital cholesteatoma of the middle ear and mastoid (a third report). Archs Otolar. *97:* 177–182 (1973).

Glasscock, M.E.; Dickins, J.R.E.; Wiet, R.: Cholesteatoma in children. Laryngoscope, St Louis *91:* 1743–1753 (1981).

Goodey, R.J.; Smyth, G.D.L.: Combined approach tympanoplasty in children. Laryngoscope, St Louis *80:* 166–171 (1970).

Jansen, C.: Cholesteatoma in children. Clin. Otolaryngol. *3:* 349–352 (1978).

Palva, A.; Karma, P.; Karja, J.: Cholesteatoma in children. Archs Otolar. *103:* 74–77 (1977).

Sanna, M.; Jemmi, G.; Bacciu, S.: La scelta della tecnica nel trattamento chirurgico del colesteatoma nell'infanzia. Annali Lar. Otol. Rinol. Faring. *75:* 1–7 (1976).

Sanna, M.; Zini, C.: Congenital cholesteatoma of the middle ear. Am. J. Otol. *5:* 368–373 (1984).

Sanna, M.; Zini, C.; Gamoletti, R.; Delogu, P.; Russo, A.; Scandellari, R.; Taibah, A.: Surgical treatment of cholesteatoma in children. Adv. Oto-Rhino-Laryng., vol. 37, pp. 110–116 (Karger, Basel 1987).

Sheehy, J.L.: Management of cholesteatoma in children. ORL *23:* 58–64 (1978).

Smyth, G.D.L.; Hassard, T.H.: Tympanoplasty in children. Am. J. Otol. *1:* 199–205 (1980).

Tos, M.: Treatment of cholesteatoma in children. A long-term study of results. Am. J. Otol. *4:* 189–197 (1983).

Zini, C.; Sanna, M.: La ricostruzione dell'apparato timpano-ossiculare nei bambini. Proc. 5th Congr. Soc. Ital. Oto-Laringol. Ped., pp. 315–338 (1980).

Mario Sanna, MD, Clinica Otorinolaringoiatrica 2°, Ospedale Maggiore, Via Gramsci 14, I–43100 Parma (Italia)

Adv. Oto-Rhino-Laryng., vol. 40, pp. 131–137 (Karger, Basel 1988)

Cholesteatoma in Children

Ph. Contencin, G. Bassereau, E. Chabardes, Y. Manac'h, Ph. Narcy

Service ORL, Hôpital Bretonneau, Faculté X Bichat, Paris, France

Middle ear cholesteatoma is a peculiarly aggressive kind of chronic otitis in children. Its fast spreading ability and its frequent trend to recurrence are well known [3, 4, 6, 14]. The actual cause of this phenomenon remains obscure although some authors think it is partially related to chronic Eustachian tube dysfunction [2].

If the treatment of this disease is generally considered as surgical [5, 11, 12], opinions differ about the technique to be used in order to eradicate the lesions with the lowest rate of recurrence and the best hearing result. The question is actually difficult when preoperative anatomy and hearing are normal and lesions widespread. Should the procedure keep the posterior canal wall intact or not?

This paper is the report of a 10-year exclusive pediatric practice in this dangerous kind of chronic otitis media.

Patients and Methods

This is a retrospective study of cases operated in the ENT/Head and Neck Surgery Department of the Bretonneau Pediatric Hospital in Paris between 1975 and 1985. Ninety-nine ears (88 patients) operated and followed up in this period represent 37% of the whole group of surgical procedures performed for chronic otitis media in the same time.

The patients' ages are shown in figure 1. There were 50 boys and 38 girls, 53 right ears, 46 left ears and 11 cases of both ears involved and operated.

The diagnosis was assessed on medical history and otoscopy. Preoperative otologic history showed interesting findings: 42 patients had already been operated. Eighteen attic openings through the external auditory canal had been performed in other institutions. This was a procedure described and advocated in France by Bourdial et al. [4] in the

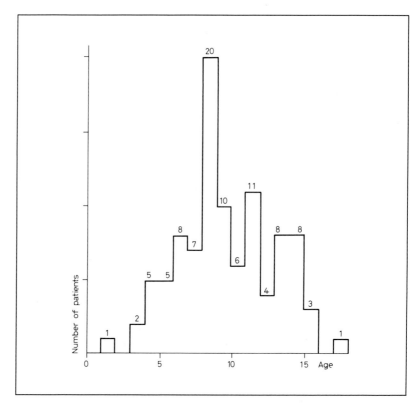

Fig. 1. Patients' age at time of surgery.

Table I. Cholesteatoma in children: preoperative history

Previous otologic procedure	42
Intrameatal attic opening	18
Ventilating tubes insertion	10
Tympanoplasty	6
ICW mastoidectomy	4
Radical mastoidectomy	2
Undetermined	2
Recurrent acute otitis media	11
Secretory otitis media	10
Cleft palate	4
Turner's syndrome	1
Renal disease	1
Heart disease	1

1950s for some simple chronic otitis, and now proved as the source of frequent iatrogenic cholesteatomas. The details of other previous otologic events are summarized in table I. Symptoms leading to medical care were ear purulent discharge in 82%, hearing loss in 13% and 5% of the cases have been discovered at the opportunity of a systematic examination. Among the few preoperative complications, we noted 2 cases of acute external mastoiditis (1 of them associated with a meningitis) and 2 cases with signs of labyrinthine fistula. No vertigo, facial paralysis, tinnitus or other symptom was observed.

Otoscopic features included 77 cases of purulent tympanic membrane perforation with accumulation of squamous epithelium, some of them with a typical polypoid mass appearing after cleaning. Nineteen cases presented as dry ears where the skin partially covered the middle ear mucosa with accumulation of debris but without any suppuration (epidermosis). Three patients had a closed tympanic membrane behind which a white mass or bulge was seen as typical aspect of 'primary' cholesteatoma.

Preoperative audiometry showed a pure conductive hearing loss with an air-bone gap from 10 to 60 db (average 35.5) in most ears. There were 4 cases of associated sensorineural hearing loss, 2 cases of normal hearing and one complete deafness.

Three main types of surgical techniques have been used in this series. The two first types are called 'open' or 'canal-down' techniques. The radical mastoidectomy mainly used until 1980 has been now abandoned for the modified mastoidectomy, with the same rules of complete eradication of osteitis, granulomatous cells and cholesteatoma with saucerization of the peripheral walls, but associated with a tympanoplasty.

The covering of the atrium mucosa with a fascia graft (over the remaining stapes or an ossiculoplasty) has been advocated to provide better anatomical and hearing results, with a dry and steady cavity [1, 7, 9, 14]. The third type of technique is a 'closed' or 'canal-up' technique which often requires a posterior tympanotomy to eradicate the cholesteatoma [5, 10–12].

In any case, a skeletonization of the dura and sigmoid sinus walls has been performed. The burr also cleans the tip of the mastoid and the retrosinusal area except in the first cases of this series where residual cholesteatoma was more frequent. A fascia graft

Table II. Anatomical classification and surgical technique

		Anatomical classification				
		I	II	III	IV	V
Otoscopy	Normal TM	–	–	1	–	2
	ME epidermosis	8	3	5	–	3
	Purulent cholesteatoma	9	6	25	10	27
Surgical techniques	'Closed'	17	6	17	1	6
	'Open'	–	3	14	9	26

Type I = Atrium; type II = attic; type III = atrium + attic; type IV = attic + mastoid; type V = atrium + attic + mastoid.

and, if necessary, an ossicular autograft or prosthesis have been used for the tympano-plasty. There were incus, malleus or bony interposition, malleus-type piston or TORP prosthesis.

Table II shows the extension of cholesteatoma found and the type of surgical proce-dure used. Thirty-seven percent of the cholesteatomas involved the mastoid, 17% were limited to the atrium.

Ossicular destruction was significantly higher regarding the incus (75% totally or partially eroded) than the stapes (35%) and the malleus (25%). Other lesions concerned the labyrinth: one fistula of the horizontal semi-circular canal and 1 case where two fistulas involved both horizontal and superior canals.

Results

The results can be considered from an anatomical and a functional point of view. Table III summarizes the rate of recurrence or residual cho-lesteatoma observed in relation to the type of surgical technique. When closed techniques have been used (ICWT), 47% of residual cholesteatomas were found, 48% in case of classical radical mastoidectomy (RM) and 18% in modified RM plus tympanoplasty.

Most of these last cases are more recent but they have a minimum follow-up of around 2 years. Residual cholesteatoma or recurrence oc-curred more frequently when the attic and the tympanic cavity were both involved (58%) than when attic (33%) or atrium (23%) alone was involved separately.

The outcome of patients who underwent an ICWT technique is the following: of the 47 cases, 17 underwent no second procedure and are followed-up as safe or cured, some for 10 years, 2 had a unique excision of small superficial 'pearl' on the tympanic membrane without any recur-rence, and 28 underwent a second surgical procedure. Of these 28 cases, 8 were safe at revision and 20 had a residual cholesteatoma. Of these 20 cases, 8 underwent a modified RM and 12 an ICWT.

Finally, of the 47 cases, 36 have a good anatomical result, 6 have been lost to follow-up (after 2 years) and 5 still present a bad result with otor-rhoea or tympanic membrane retraction. Including the cases who under-went an open technique and excluding the patients lost to follow-up, of 77 patients, we note 67 good anatomical results, 4 tympanic membrane anom-alies (retraction or perforation) and 6 persistent otorrhoea to be operated again.

Table IV summarizes the audiometry results under the shape of the average pure tone air-conduction thresholds. On the right of the table, one

Table III. Rate of recurrence related to surgery technique and period

	1975–1980		1981–1985		Total	
	n	%	n	%	n	%
CT	13/23	56	9/24	37	22/47	47
RM	13/27	48	1/2	50	14/29	48
RMT	2/5	40	2/18	11	4/23	18
Total	28/55	51	12/44	27	40/99	40

CT = 'Closed technique'; RM = radical mastoidectomy; RMT = radical mastoidectomy + tympanoplasty.

Table IV. Mean audiometry aerial thresholds related to stapes status

	Safe stapes (n = 67)			Destroyed stapes (n = 32)			Total (n = 99)		
	CT	RM	RMT	CT	RM	RMT	CT	RM	RMT
Preoperative	28	47	40	28	37	47	28	42	42
					1 coph				
Postoperative	22	44	30	33	44	45	23	44	35
					2 coph				

can note the improvement of the thresholds in case of closed technique (28–23 dB), the slight deterioration in case of radical mastoidectomy (42–44 dB) and the improvement in case of modified RM plus tympanoplasty (42–35 dB). On the left of the table, one can see the results are much better when the stapes is intact.

The post-operative audiometry repartition of patients is interesting to consider: 31 cases (39%) have an air-conduction average threshold better than 30 dB (which always corresponds, in our audiometry results, to an air-bone gap inferior or equal to 20 dB). Thirty-two (40%) are in the 30- to 50-dB range and 17 (21%) remain with a bad hearing result. We have noted 2 cases of cophosis who presented with a labyrinthine fistula.

Discussion

This study confirms the classical data of the literature concerning cholesteatoma in children: generally easy diagnosis at otoscopy for the otologist, necessity of surgical treatment without any delay, heavy trend to recurrence.

Fortunately, complications seem to remain rare in our countries and for this part of population.

As most authors reported [2, 8, 11, 14], the choice of the surgical technique depends on preoperative hearing, size of the mastoid and lesions spread but also, mainly for us, on age and estimated feasibility of a long, long follow-up. In fact, our patient population is largely constituted of immigrants and worker families, which frequently leave the area. As Abramson [2] noted in 1985 'Patient compliance is not always easy to ensure, since the original decision is made primarily with parents and not with the patient'. We hold the same attitude and we replaced the closed technique by radical mastoidectomy, alone first, then with tympanoplasty. With this last technique, we observed a smaller rate of residual cholesteatoma and acceptable hearing results.

Therefore, our present attitude is now the following; we perform a closed technique only if: (1) lesions are limited and easy to eradicate through an ICWT with a posterior tympanotomy; (2) the ossicular chain is undamaged; (3) there is a reliable family context for a long follow-up, and (4) a second procedure is planned 8–18 months later.

If one of these conditions is lacking, we perform a modified radical mastoidectomy plus tympanoplasty. And if no infectious lesion is left in the mastoid and under repeated postoperative care with drops and suction, a dry and steady cavity is obtained.

References

1   Abramson, M.; Lachenbuch, P.A.; Press, B.H.; McCabe, B.F.: Results of conservative surgery for middle ear cholesteatoma. Laryngoscope *87:* 1281–1287 (1977).
2   Abramson, M.: Open or closed tympanomastoidectomy for cholesteatoma in children. Am. J. Otol. *6:* 167–169 (1985).
3   Andrieu-Guitrancourt, J.; Dehesdin, D.; Schlosser, M.: Traitement de l'otite moyenne chronique cholestéatomateuse de l'enfant. Annls Oto-lar. *97:* 39–44 (1980).
4   Bourdial, J.; Debain, J.J.; Coussieux, P.; Lallemant, Y.: L'otite chronique de l'enfant. Rapport du congrès de la Société Française d'ORL (Arnette, Paris 1955).

5   Charachon, R.; Gratacap, B.: The surgical treatment of cholesteatoma in children. Clin. Otolar. *10:* 177–184 (1985).
6   Cody, D.T.R.; Taylor, W.F.: Mastoidectomy for acquired cholesteatoma. Long-term results. First international conference on cholesteatoma, pp. 337–351 (Aesculapius, New York 1977).
7   Cody, D.T.; Macdonald, T.J.: Mastoidectomy for acquired cholesteatoma. Follow up to 20 years. Laryngoscope *94:* 1027–1030 (1984).
8   Glasscock, M.E.; Dickens, J.R.E.; Wiet, R.: Cholesteatoma in children. Laryngoscope *91:* 1743–1753 (1981).
9   Fleury, P.; Basset, J.M.; Brasnu, D.; Compere, J.F.; Pansier, P.: L'évidement: tabou de l'otite chronique cholestéatomateuse. Annls Oto-lar. *97:* 35–38 (1980).
10 Palva, A.; Karma, P.; Karja, J.: Cholesteatoma in children. Archs Otol. *103:* 74–77 (1977).
11 Sheehy, J.L.: Cholesteatoma surgery in children. Am. J. Otol. *6:* 170–172 (1985).
12 Smyth, G.D.L.: Cholesteatoma surgery: the influence of the canal wall. Laryngoscope *95:* 92–96 (1985).
13 Tomioka, S.; Iino, Y.; Yuasa, R.; Saijo, S.; Kaneko, Y.: Clinical observation of middle ear cholesteatoma in children; in Kultura, Proc. 4th Int. Congr. Pediatric Otolaryngology, Budapest, in press.
14 Wayoff, M.; Charachon, R.; Roulleau, P.; Lacher, G.; Deguine, C.: Le traitement chirurgical du cholestéatome de l'oreille moyenne. Rapport à la Société Française d'ORL (Arnette, Paris 1982).

Ph. Contencin, MD, Service ORL, Hôpital Bretonneau, Faculté X. Bichat, 2, rue Carpeaux, F-75877 Paris Cédex 18 (France)

Adv. Oto-Rhino-Laryng., vol. 40, pp. 138–141 (Karger, Basel 1988)

Open Cavity Mastoidectomy in Children

Hearing Results at 5 Years

T.H. Guerrier

Ear, Nose and Throat Department, Royal Hampshire County Hospital,
Winchester, Hampshire, UK

Introduction

After the radical open cavity operation had been established by Viennese otologists, it was the standard operation for cholesteatoma for 40 years. The operation produced a safe ear, but at a cost: a discharging cavity and deafness in a large number of cases.

In the late 1950s, Claus Jansen introduced a new concept with the closed cavity operation: by retaining the essential anatomy, the open cavity was avoided and the prospects for functional repair greatly improved. However, it has since been shown by many eminent otologists that the operation is technically difficult and should be staged (table I).

The last 20 years have seen many publications arguing the relative merits of the two approaches to the problem of cholesteatoma. The attention has been rightly focussed on recurrent or residual disease, but there have been very few reports of long-term hearing results. Gordon Smyth's meticulous long-term studies are unique, but would suggest that the hope for good long-term hearing from the closed cavity operation has not been wholly fulfilled.

Was the open cavity operation really so bad? How much of the success of the closed cavity operation was due to its design philosophy, and how much to better otological surgery in general?

Materials and Methods

This paper presents a consecutive series of children with cholesteatoma operated on by the open cavity method. All have been followed for a minimum of 5 years. All were under 11 years at operation. All had extensive cholesteatoma, many with erosion of the

Table I.

Open cavity operation	Closed cavity operation
1 operation	2 or more operations
Simple	Difficult
Discharge	Dry
Poor hearing	Good hearing

dura of the middle and posterior cranial fossae. All the ears in this series had ossicular discontinuity but a mobile stapes.

There was nothing original in the operative technique. Many were performed by a registrar of average experience, and all were one-stage procedures. All ears were treated by local antibiotics to obtain as dry an ear as possible. The operation was a standard modified radical mastoidectomy. The middle ear repair was to insert an autologous bone chip as a malleus stapes assembly. Sometimes this repair was unstable, then the chip would be placed on the head of the stapes with a portion tucked under the handle of the malleus. The tympanic membrane was augmented by temporalis fascia. The whole repair was supported by a gelatin sponge. Tissue glues were not used in this series. Because of the extensive nature of the cholesteatoma in so many of these children, and the doubt about their reliability in attending for long-term review, no attempt was made to obliterate the mastoid bowl in this series.

Discussion

There are 42 ears in the series. Forty have maintained dry, stable cavities over 5 years. The other two developed severe retraction of the lower part of the tympanic membrane into the hypotympanum, with mucous membrane developing on the outer surface. Neither child has opted for a review operation, the ear being kept dry with occasional local attention (table II).

Thirty-four ears have maintained an air-bone gap of less than 10 dB over 5 years. This figure of 80% compares well with the figures for the closed cavity operation given by Smith.

The 2 wet ears have hearing losses at 50–60 dB, as might have been expected. Both children have good hearing in the other ear, and both ears operated on were deaf to about 50–60 dB before the operation.

Of the other failures, 2 had air-bone gap closure 3 months after the operation, but the prosthesis had slipped in each ear. Each ear now has an

Table II.

Number of ears	Air-bone gap, dB	Causes of failure
34	10	
2	50–60	mucous membrane lining meatus
2	35–40	Slipped prosthesis
1	35–40	fibrosis
1	20–25	graft extrusion
2	35–40	'fibrosis'

air-bone gap of 35–40 dB. Because the hearing is good in the opposite ear, and there is no apparent education handicap, these 2 ears have not been reexplored.

One ear had extensive granulations in the middle ear cleft at operation. A disc of silastic was placed in the ear to maintain the air space, but although the ear appears to have some ventilation, the hearing never improved satisfactorily. The postoperative result gave an air-bone gap of 25 dB, which has declined slowly over 6 years to 35–40 dB. This is the preoperative figure for that ear.

One ear has partially extruded the autologous bone chip. The hearing was good initially, with an air-bone gap of 10–15 dB. The tympanic membrane repair then became thinner and thinner. It was thought that it would break down altogether; but it has held up only to wrap itself over the partially extruded prosthesis. The hearing declined over the first year to settle at an air-bone gap of 20–25 dB. This is an improvement on the pre-operative hearing of 40 dB. Again because the hearing is good in the opposite ear, and there is no educational handicap, the ear has not been reexplored.

The last two ears are disappointing. Both were dry at operation, while cholesteatoma was extensive in both ears. This applied to all the ears in this series. Both operations were technically straightforward, and both children had uneventful recoveries. The initial hearing results were fairly good at 15 dB, but the hearing has slowly slipped to the present figure of 40 dB in 1 case, and 35 dB in the other. This represents the preoperative hearing in each case.

The hearing has not been made worse in any ear in this series. 34 of 42 ears have maintained good hearing for a minimum of 5 years. One additional child has better hearing than before operation, although only at 20–25 dB. She feels that her hearing in the play-ground has improved, although she says that she has noticed no improvement in school classes.

These results of a consecutive series of ears with extensive cholesteatoma, discontinuity of the ossicular chain, but an intact stapes show better hearing than one would expect from the open-cavity operation. Why? I suspect that I have been lucky. A high proportion of the children came from poor social backgrounds. The families have recently been rehoused from the London slums to new houses built on the edge of towns and villages near Winchester. Perhaps the original living conditions predisposed to the development of chronic ear disease. Perhaps the new conditions predispose to healthy ears.

T.H. Guerrier, FRCS, Ear, Nose and Throat Department, Royal Hampshire County Hospital, Winchester, Hampshire, Winchester SO22 5DG (UK)

Adv. Oto-Rhino-Laryng., vol. 40, pp. 142–148 (Karger, Basel 1988)

Treatment of Cholesteatoma in Children

Residual Cholesteatoma Related to Observation Time

Mirko Tos, Torben Lau

ENT Department, Gentofte University Hospital, Hellerup, Denmark

Introduction

Surgeons employing the intact canal wall technique for cholesteatoma consistently perform second-look operations in children; the rate of residual cholesteatoma reported by these surgeons range from 27 to 61% [1–4]. All of our cholesteatoma surgery is carried out in one stage and at follow-up we find residual cholesteatoma in 10% of the ears [5]. This large discrepancy in the rate of residual cholesteatomas may be due to the fact that these are not detected without a second-look operation. However, with increasing observation time, one would expect the residue to grow and at some stage become visible. Our series of children with cholesteatoma has been subjected to several follow-up examinations, which makes it possible for us to analyze the increase in recurrence rate with increasing observation time, and this is the object of the present study.

Material and Method

During a period of 14 years (1965 through 1978), 120 children (122 ears), aged 2–14 years, underwent surgery for cholesteatoma. There were 41 ears with attic cholesteatoma with retraction (perforation) of Shrapnell's membrane; 57 ears with sinus cholesteatoma and posterosuperior retraction (perforation), and 24 ears with tensa retraction cholesteatoma with retraction of the whole pars tensa. 25% of the sinus cholesteatomas and 33% of the tensa retraction cholesteatomas were localized exclusively in the tympanic cavity, whereas the remaining extended either to the attic or the antrum.

All operations were performed in one stage. In 26 ears with sinus or tensa retraction cholesteatomas confined to the tympanic cavity, the cholesteatoma was removed by tympanoplasty without mastoidectomy. During the period 1965–1971, 45 ears underwent canal down mastoidectomy, reconstruction of the ear canal, and obliteration of the cavity. From 1972 to 1978, 51 ears received a modified canal wall up mastoidectomy [6, 7]. The ossicular chain was intact in 15% of the ears, the incus was defective in 57%, and the stapedial arch was lacking in 27 ears. The materials used for interposition between the stapes and the eardrum and as columella between the footplate and the eardrum included auto- and homologous ossicles, and autologous cortical bone. A temporal muscle fascia was used for closure of tympanic membrane perforations and reconstruction of the ear canal.

Results

The results of the individual procedures have previously been described in detail, just as the pros and cons of canal wall up and canal wall down mastoidectomy have been analyzed [7]. We present here the alterations in the results occurring with increasing observation time.

Observation Time

The patients were reexamined regularly up to 2 years postoperatively; the results at the last examination during this period are denoted as the primary results. After this period the patients were reexamined 6 times by the authors (in 1968, 1972, 1976, 1978, 1980/81 and 1985/86), and the last examination forms the basis for the late results. Median observation time was 9.5 years, range 3–21 years, and 98% of the children were reexamined at least once. Owing to the great number of reexaminations, of which several took place already during the collection of the material, we obtained a high follow-up rate and were able to reduce the difference between the theoretically longest observation time and the actual observation time (table I). Thus, patients who did not attend the last follow-up examination had participated in one of the preceding ones.

Recurrence and Observation Time

At the follow-up examination in 1985/86, a total of 13 (11%) residual cholesteatomas had been found in the tympanic cavity and 2 (2%) in the attic. In addition, 6 (5%) recurrent cholesteatomas were found in the attic or antrum. The corresponding values at the follow-up examination carried out in 1980/81 were 8, 2 and 2%, respectively; in all, 5% fewer than in 1985/86.

Most of the residual cholesteatomas were found during the first 5 years (fig. 1). After the 8th postoperative year we have not encountered any

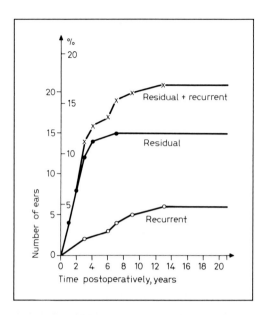

Fig. 1. Cumulative increase of residual and recurrent cholesteatomas with increasing observation time.

residual cholesteatomas in spite of the fact that more than 13% of the ears had an observation time exceeding 15 years and 43% exceeding 10 years (table I). Recurrent cholesteatomas were detected and removed up to 14 years after the first procedure; they all developed in the cavity following canal down mastoidectomy.

Most cholesteatomas were detected at follow-up (table II), either in discharging ears or in ears with a progressing retraction that could not be surveyed. Only a few, small cholesteatomas were found in the tympanic cavity at operation for hearing impairment.

Reoperations

Although our policy has been to reoperate on as few ears as possible, a total of 40 ears (33%) required a second procedure, and of these 10 needed two reoperations. Reoperation was performed either because of cholesteatoma or because ossiculoplasty was required (table III).

By far the majority of patients underwent reoperation during the first 2 postoperative years, but some were reoperated on more than 10 years after the first procedure.

Table I. Number of ears with longest possible (optimal) postoperative observation time related to definite observation time

Optimal observation time, years	Number of ears	Definite observation time, years				
		>15	11–15	6–10	3–5	<2
>15	33	16	8	8	1	
11–15	51		28	15	8	
6–10	38			27	9	2
Total	122	16	36	50	18	2

Table II. When and how the recurrent cholesteatomas were detected

Detected	Time after the first operation, years				Total	
	0.5–2	3–5	6–10	>10	n	%
Detected at control (without symptoms)	2	3	–	–	5	2
Suspected at control (discharge)	5	4	2	1	12	12
Unexpected (reoperation for hearing loss)	1	1	2	–	4	2.5
Total until 1985/86	8	8	4	1	21	17
Total until 1980/81	8	5	–	1	14	12

Table III. Cause and time of reoperation

Cause of reoperation	Time of reoperation, years				Total	
	0.5–2	3–5	6–10	11–15	n	%
Residual cholesteatoma	8	6	1	–	15	12
Recurrent cholesteatoma	–	2	2	1	5	4
Ossiculoplasty	6	3	2	1	12	10
Cavity problems	–	–	2	–	2	2
Reperforation	1	2	–	2	5	4
Deep retraction	1	–	–	–	1	1
Total	16	13	7	4	40	33

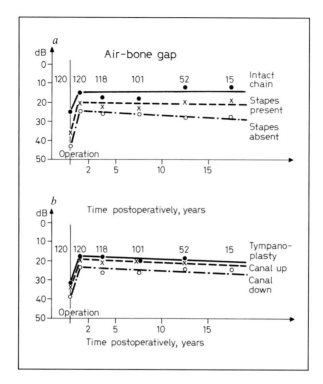

Fig. 2. Cholesteatoma in children. *a* Mean air-bone gaps preoperatively and in different postoperative periods in ears with intact ossicular chain, ears with stapes present, and ears with stapes absent. *b* Mean air-bone gap in ears with tympanoplasty only, ears with canal wall up and canal down mastoidectomy. Hearing was evaluated in only 120 ears.

At the last follow-up, 5% of the ears had eardrum perforations, 7% had tympanosclerosis, 15% displayed a partially or completely adherent eardrum, and 12% had thickened and rigid eardrums. Secretory otitis was present in only 1% of the ears and a completely normal and mobile pars tensa could be demonstrated in 60% of the ears.

Hearing and Observation Time

Our many follow-up examinations permit us to analyze alterations in the air-bone gap (in the frequency range 500–2,000 Hz) with increasing observation time (fig. 2a). The best and most stable postoperative air-bone gaps were found in ears with intact ossicular chain. As expected, the poorest results and those declining most markedly over the years were obtained in ears lacking the stapedial arch.

Hearing was best in ears receiving tympanoplasty without mastoidectomy (fig. 2b). There was a tendency toward better postoperative results in ears undergoing canal up mastoidectomy compared with ears with canal down mastoidectomy. The latter group, however, also had the poorest air-bone gaps preoperatively.

Discussion and Conclusion

The vast majority of children with residual cholesteatoma and recurrent cholesteatoma had local symptoms, and the residue was detected at a clinical examination. Undetected residual cholesteatomas must be expected over a period of 10 years to grow so much so as to draw attention to themselves. Therefore, we do not feel it is necessary to perform second-stage operations in order to detect residual cholesteatomas. Another argument brought forward in defence of second-stage operations is that the functional results are better. As second-stage operations entail a considerably larger number of procedures than do one-stage procedures, the total functional results ought to be better than can be obtained with a smaller number of operations. Whether or not this is the case has never been documented, especially not with regard to the long-term results. Planned two-stage operations, however, do not solve all the problems that may arise over a long period of observation, including cavity problems, late reperforation, and hearing impairment as well as problems caused by late ossicular fixation and late retractions or by poor tubal function.

In accord with our previous analyses of results in children, this study shows that canal wall up as well as canal wall down mastoidectomy have their place in the treatment of children's cholesteatoma. In adhesive ears with poor tubal function, canal down mastoidectomy is preferable; in ears with a large mastoid cell system and a relatively air-filled tympanic cavity, canal wall up mastoidectomy has proved by far to be the best method, especially in view of the fact that cavities in children can be problematic. If the cholesteatoma mass is confined to the tympanic cavity, our preference is tympanoplasty without mastoidectomy.

References

1   Sheehy, J.L.: Cholesteatoma surgery in children. Acta oto-rhino-lar. *34:* 98–106 (1980).
2   Charachon, P.; Gratacap, B.: The surgical treatment of cholesteatoma in children. Clin. Otolaryngol. *10:* 177–184 (1985).
3   Jahnke, V.; Falk, W.: Zur Klinik, Pathologie und Behandlung des Cholesteatoma im Kindesalter. Lar. Rhinol. *55:* 556–560 (1976).
4   Smyth, G.D.L.: Postoperative cholesteatoma in combined approach tympanoplasty. J. Lar. Otol. *90:* 597–621 (1976).
5   Tos, M.: Treatment of cholesteatoma in children. A long-term study of results. Am. J. Otol. *4:* 189–197 (1982).
6   Tos, M.: Obliteration of the cavity in mastoidectomy. Acta oto-lar. *67:* 516–520 (1969).
7   Tos, M.: Cholesteatoma in children. Am. J. Otol. (in press, 1987).

M. Tos, MD, ENT Department, Gentofte University Hospital,
DK–2900 Hellerup (Denmark)

Adv. Oto-Rhino-Laryng., vol. 40, pp. 149–155 (Karger, Basel 1988)

Tympanoplasty as Surgical Treatment of Cholesteatoma in Children

R. Charachon, B. Gratacap

Clinique Universitaire ORL du CHU de Grenoble, Grenoble, France

Introduction

Cholesteatoma is usually very extensive in children. There are two possible explanations: the speed of tissue growth and the degree of infection and inflammation brought by the Eustachian tube. The cholesteatoma develops rapidly in a pneumatized mastoid which it takes by surprise. All these factors explain the extensive, finger-like shape taken by cholesteatoma in children.

Surgical treatment has to avoid 3 pitfalls: (1) a large cavity left by the open technique in a well-pneumatized mastoid; (2) a residual cholesteatoma in the closed technique or entrapped behind the flap of the obliteration technique, and (3) a retraction pocket produced by tubal dysfunction.

Materials and Methods

We reviewed 159 cholesteatomas in children. Surgery was performed by the first author between 1966 and 1984. Previously, we reported the results of surgery on 141 cholesteatomas in children performed between 1966 and 1981 in our department by different surgeons [1]. Cholesteatomas were bilateral in 11 cases and 10 were discovered behind an intact tympanic membrane. External semicircular canal fistula was rare. A fixed stapes, sometimes only at the second stage, was seen fairly frequently (11 and 1 bilateral). The arch of the stapes was very often destroyed (46%).

Pathological Findings

In spite of medical treatment (topical and systemic antibiotics, repeated suctions) purulent discharge was present at the operation in 39% of the cases. Three children had an extensive cholesteatoma in the weak point of the retrotympanum below the sinus tympani, deep to the facial nerve. This area is approached between the lateral sinus and facial nerve below the posterior semicircular canal. This opening is checked at the second stage. In one of these cases, it was possible to explore between the facial nerve and the posterior semicircular canal with a small diamond burr (0.8 mm) and to approach the sinus tympani from behind.

Another cholesteatoma extension is sometimes found into the anterosuperior cell tract above the tympanic portion of the facial nerve and anterior to the superior semicircular canal. It is necessary to identify the facial nerve and superior canal after removing the incus and malleus head and opening the supratubal recess.

Sometimes, the posterosuperior cell tract is invaded between the dural plates and the superior semicircular canal. In addition to this series, we had to operate on a temporal bone cholesteatoma in a child of 15.

Surgical Procedures

Radical Mastoidectomy. This technique consists of joining the tympanic cavity and the mastoid into one single cavity be removing the posterosuperior part of the bony canal. All overhangs must be eliminated as anterior and posterior buttress of the attic. Edges of the cavity must be properly shaped (Paparella's saucerization). A meatoplasty is performed according to the size of the cavity.

Open Technique Tympanoplasty. This is very similar to radical mastoidectomy, the only difference is rebuilding of the tympanic membrane and a simple columella.

Obliteration Technique (fig. 1). We used this procedure since 1966 with a superior and/or posterior flap and since 1973 with a Palva flap. Staging was performed to improve initially functional results when the mesotympanum was dissected. Staging is now used in a few cases to check posterior cavities behind the flap.

A posterosuperior approach is performed. A Palva flap is prepared with all the musculo-periosteal tissue covering the mastoid and left attached to the edge of the concha. A 'traction meatoplasty' is prepared comprising 3 steps: a skin resection of a part of posterosuperior approach, an incision between the tragus and the helix dividing the anterior limit of the Palva flap, and, at the end of the operation, a slightly tense suture on two levels opening the incision between tragus and helix.

Radical mastoidectomy is performed with saucerization of the margins of the cavity. The bony canal wall is lowered to the level of the floor of the ear canal and to the level of the facial nerve. If the sinus tympani is involved, the facial nerve is skeletonized. Cholesteatoma is very carefully dissected and again drilling is performed where it is necessary. If the mesotympanum is covered by safe mucosa, and if the stapes is intact, it is possible to do only one stage. The tympanic membrane is reconstructed usually with fascia in underlay. A homograft of the malleus head is inserted on the stapes. The obliteration is carried out by free fibromuscular grafts in attic and antrum covered by the fibromuscular flap. The fascia graft rests on the flap. The canal skin is finally folded back over the flap and the graft. If the mesotympanum has been dissected raw, or if the crura are missing, a silastic sheeting is placed in the mesotympanum to prevent adhesion and a second stage is performed 12 months later through the meatus. A tympanoparietal flap is cut in the muscle obliteration. The silastic sheeting is removed and the ossicular chain is reconstructed. In rare cases, the flap itself is partially lifted during the second stage. The posterior approach

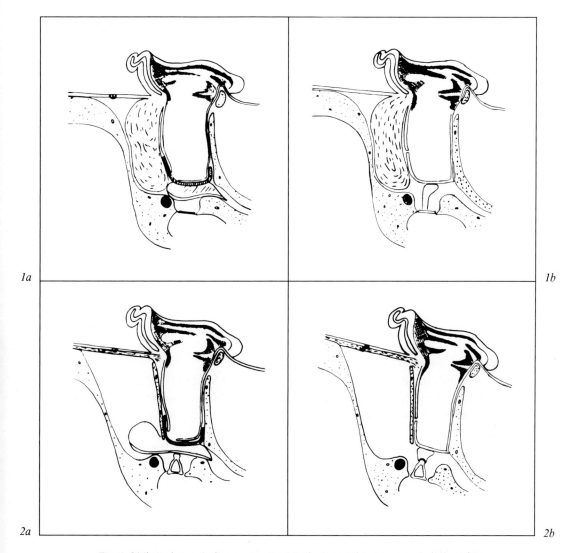

1a *1b* *2a* *2b*

Fig. 1. Obliteration technique. *a* 1st stage: radical mastoidectomy – rebuilding of the tympanic membrane with a fascia graft, obliteration of the posterior cavity with a Palva flap, traction meatoplasty, silastic sheeting if necessary. *b* 2nd stage: 12 months later, through the meatus, removal of silastic and rebuilding of the ossicular chain, sometimes a checking of the posterior cavity by posterior approach and by partial lifting of the flap.

Fig. 2. Intact canal wall techique. *a* 1st stage: posterior tympanotomy, fascia graft as an underlay, closure of any attic defect using thin tragal cartilage with its perichondrium, insertion of silastic sheeting. *b* 2nd stage: 18 months later, checking of all the middle ear and rebuilding of the ossicular chain.

is used to lift the flap from the mastoid, antrum and aditus. The flap must be left attached to the external semicircular canal and area of the mastoid part of the facial nerve.

Closed Technique (fig. 2). Initially, this operation has been performed in one stage. Since 1973 it has been staged systematically. At the first stage, the cholesteatoma is removed with preservation of the bony canal and posterior tympanotomy. An initial separation of the incudo-stapedial joint is done in case the incus is intact to prevent high-tone deafness due to contact of the burr with ossicular chain. The tympanic membrane is rebuilt with fascia usually as an underlay and silastic sheeting is inserted into the middle ear. If there is an attic defect, it is carefully closed using thin cartilage with its perichondrium.

At the second stage, 18–24 months later, the silastic sheeting is removed by a new posterior approach. The whole middle ear is carefully checked. If a cholesteatoma cyst is found, it is removed with the surrounding mucosa. The ossicular chain is rebuilt. If the stapes is intact, an incus homograft or malleus head is placed vertically between the head of the stapes and the tympanic membrane. In such a case, this reconstruction is sometimes performed at the first stage. If the stapes crura are absent, we prefer to reconstruct the ossicular chain by using an autograft tragal cartilage if stiff enough, or a total incus homograft, or sometimes a ceravital Torp® prosthesis.

Results

Anatomical

The rate of follow-up is 66% at 5 years and 50% at 10 years. *An intact tympanic membrane* was achieved between 89 (obliteration technique, 1st stage with silastic) and 100% of the time (closed technique and obliteration technique in one stage).

Residual cholesteatoma (table I) may be studied only in the two-stage tympanoplasties. The incidence of residual cholesteatoma was about the same in the closed (31%) as in the obliteration technique (38%). These residual cholesteatoma were carefully removed. In 3 cases of the closed technique with 2 cysts, a third stage was done 2 years later finding healthy mucosa in 2 cases and a small cyst in the 3rd. In one case of the closed technique, a large cholesteatoma was found in the attic and the mesotympanum and an obliteration technique was performed at the 2nd stage.

The incidence of *retraction pockets* (table II) is very low in the obliteration technique. Nevertheless, we observed one retraction pocket eroding a lateral semicircular canal fistula in 1 case 10 years after an obliteration technique in 2 stages. In the closed technique, an interesting figure is observed during a follow-up of 10 years. In the one-stage closed technique, a retraction pocket occurred in 20% of the cases. In the two-stage closed technique, a retraction pocket occurred in 12.5% of cases after the 1st stage, and 7.5% after the 2nd (i.e. 20% for all closed techniques in 2 stages!). When a retraction pocket is observed at the second stage of a closed technique, an obliteration technique is performed.

Table I. Children cholesteatoma: 1966–1984, residual cholesteatomas removed at second stages

Closed technique = 29/93 (31%) (ICWT)		
Small cyst tympanic membrane	2	4 cases with 2 cysts
Mesotympanum	13	1 mesotympanum + Eustachian tube
Attic	9	2 mesotympanum + tympanic membrane
Eustachian tube	0	1 mesotympanum + attic
Mastoid	0	→ 3 third stages
Larger cholesteatoma attic + mesotympanum → MOT		
Obliteration technique = 10/26 (38%) (MOT)		
Small cyst antrum	1	
Epitympanum	3	
Mesotympanum	5	
Tympanic membrane	1	

Table II. Children cholesteatoma: 1966–1984, retraction pockets

Closed technique (ICWT)	One stage 14		3 years	1 → MOT	20%
			5 years	1 → MOT	
			10 years	1 → MOT	
	Two stages	After 1st stage (96)	1 year	12 → MOT	12.5%
		After 2nd stage (80)	4 months	1 followed	7.5%
			1 year	1 → ICWT	
				1 → MOT	
				1 ?	
			3 years	1 → MOT	
				1 followed	
Obliteration technique (MOT)	One stage 16				
	Two stages	After 1st stage (27)		0	
		After 2nd stage (26)	10 years	1 → MOT (ESC fistula)	
		After ICWT		0	

Anatomical failures after planned surgery may be compared between unstaged and staged cases. In the unstaged closed techniques, besides retraction pockets, one cholesteatoma in the mesotympanum had to be revised. In the obliteration techniques, one mesotympanum fibrosis underwent 3 revisions without any result and an attic cholesteatoma was treated by an open technique.

In the staged closed techniques, besides retraction pockets already studied, we observed seromucous otitis 3 times. Three intratympanic cholesteatomas and one mesotympanum cholesteatoma had to be revised. In staged obliteration techniques, besides one retraction pocket already studied, we observed a cholesteatoma between skin and flap producing a narrowed external canal.

Hearing

They were studied only when the footplate or the stapes were mobile. In 4 cases of a mesotympanum cholesteatoma, an *intact ossicular chain* was preserved with good result.

When the stapes was intact, the air-conduction threshold was between 0 and 30 dB in 55% of cases and the air-bone gap between 0 and 20 dB in 64% of cases with results slightly better in the one-stage closed technique.

When the stapes crura were absent, the air-conduction threshold was between 0 and 30 dB in 37% of the cases and the air-bone gap between 0 and 20 dB in 34% of the cases. The results were slightly better in two stages.

The sensorineural impairment was calculated as the average loss at 4 and 8 kHz before and after surgery. We found a loss between 20 and 40 dB in 10 cases and between 40 and 60 dB in 1 case. A second case of important loss was observed after 3 attempts of functional revision in a case of mesotympanum fibrosis (obliteration technique in one stage).

Conclusions

An intact canal wall technique with a facial recess opening in 2 stages has priority in children because the mastoid is well pneumatized and the cholesteatoma is large. This technique avoids a large cavity and a second stage allows removal of small residual cholesteatomas. If an early retraction pocket or a large residual cholesteatoma is found at the second stage, the intact canal wall technique must be converted into an obliteration technique.

An obliteration technique with a Palva flap as first procedure is safe only if there is no risk of cholesteatoma remaining behind the flap. This procedure is reserved for small cholesteatomas in a narrow sclerotic mastoid and is of great value in cholesteatomas limited to the mesotympanum. In any case, undermining must be very careful and completed by drilling all surfaces of the mastoid. Staging with silastic sheeting is used only if the mesotympanum needs to be dissected. A revision of the flap is possible.

An open technique is used when mastoiditis with an abscess is present. Radical mastoidectomy is still the best procedure for intracranial complications.

Reference

1   Charachon, R.; Gratacap, B.: The surgical treatment of cholesteatoma in children. Clin. Otolaryngol. *10:* 177–184 (1985).

R. Charachon, MD, Clinique Universitaire ORL du CHU de Grenoble, BP 217X, F–38043 Grenoble Cedex (France)

Adv. Oto-Rhino-Laryng., vol. 40, pp. 156–161 (Karger, Basel 1988)

When To Do Tympanoplasty in Children?

Torben Lau, Mirko Tos

ENT Department, Gentofte University Hospital, Hellerup, Denmark

Introduction

There is a general agreement that children with cholesteatoma should undergo surgery as soon as possible, regardless of age. In contrast, the question of when to treat non-cholesteatomatous chronic otitis, and in particular when to close a dry perforation of the tympanic membrane, is much debated. When shall you close a dry perforation? Not at pre-school age? Not before the child has reached the age of 10 or 14 years? Shall tympanoplasty in children be very restricted? or can it be done at any age? If the ear is discharging: Shall you perform a mastoidectomy first, and then tympanoplasty in a second stage? Or shall you do a one-stage procedure with an intact canal wall mastoidectomy and tympanoplasty? By this study we will give our contribution to this debate.

Different authors have found different graft-take rates; from 53% by Bluestone et al. [1], who find that children are not good candidates for tympanoplasty, to 90% by Smyth and Hassard [2], who recommend tympanoplasty as soon as possible. Gans [3] and Kleinfeldt et al. [4] have found a poorer healing in children than in adults, but recommend operation anyhow, because of increasing pathology of the ossicular chain by age. Buchwald and Birck [5] have found reperforations in 34% 1 year after surgery. Raine and Singh [6] have shown that the graft-take success improves with increasing age. We, in this study, have found a graft-take rate at 92%, and we do recommend tympanoplasty in children of all ages.

Material and Method

From 1968 to 1980 tympanoplasty was performed in 124 ears in 116 children with non-cholesteatomatous chronic otitis. Twenty-six of the children were 2–7 years old, the rest were 8–14 years old. Ninety-four had sequelae to otitis, most of them with a dry perforation of the tympanic membrane. Twenty-two had granulating otitis; 12 of these ears were treated with an additional canal wall down mastoidectomy, and 7 were treated with an additional canal wall up mastoidectomy. Eight ears had adhesive otitis.

The ossicular chain was intact in 69%. Twenty-six percent had a defected incus, but an intact stapes arcade. Only 5% had a defected stapes suprastructure. One hundred and twelve ears (90%) had perforations of the tympanic membrane. In 20% the perforations were located anteriorly, in 21% inferiorly, and in 19% posteriorly. In 22% the perforation was total. The myringoplasty was done as on-lay, except in ears with posteriorly located perforations, where it was done as under-lay. The middle ear mucosa was normal in 56% of the ears, thickened in 11%, granulating in 14%, and secretory in 19%.

We did a follow-up investigation 3–15 years after surgery. Median follow-up time was 7 years. Eighty-nine percent joined the investigation. Those that did not join the follow-up investigation, did not differ in any respect preoperatively or primarily after surgery, from those that *did* join the follow-up.

Results

Reperforations

We found reperforations occurring primarily (within 2 years after surgery) in 7 ears (6%). Six of those 7 ears were reoperated, and 5 of them with success. Thus, 2 years after surgery, there were only reperforations in 2 ears. One of these 2 ears did not join the follow-up, the other still had a perforation at the last evaluation, in addition we found new perforations in 3 more ears, and during the observation time 1 ear developed a reperforation and was reoperated with success elsewhere. Thus, in total, reperforations developed in 11 ears (9%) (fig. 1). There was no difference between the youngest and the eldest age groups according to reperforations. Two out of 26 ears (8%) had reperforations in the youngest group, and 9 out of 98 ears (9%) had reperforations in the eldest group.

Hearing

The hearing results were satisfactory. Seventy-one percent had a hearing gain more than 10 dB, both primarily and at the last evaluation. We found a closing of the air-bone gap to 20 dB or better in 88%, compared to 27% preoperatively. We found a speech reception threshold (SRT) of 30 dB or better in 88% compared to 58% preoperatively (table I). There was no difference in the results obtained in children 2–7 years old, compared to the results obtained in children 8–14 years old. An absolute hearing level of 30 dB or better was found in 88% of the children in both groups, and a closing of the air-bone to 20 dB or less was obtained in 88% of the younger

Table I. Hearing preoperatively and primarily in 124 ears, and at the last examination 3–15 years post-operatively in 110 ears

	Absolute hearing, %		SRT, %		Air-bone gap, %			Hearing gain (in dB), %				
	0–20 dB	0–30 dB	0–20 dB	0–30 dB	0–10 dB	0–20 dB	0–30 dB	> 20 dB	> 10 dB	1–10 dB	no gain in dB	deteriorated in dB
Preoperatively	19	43	27	56	5	27	60	–	–	–	–	–
Primarily	64	87	81	90	48	80	93	27	71	20	4	5
Late	74	88	76	88	56	88	97	41	71	18	6	5

Frequency range 500–2,000 Hz. Four methods of evaluation: Absolute hearing level, air-bone gap, SRT (speech reception threshold) and hearing gain.

Table II. Absolute hearing and air-bone gap preoperatively and postoperatively (primarily and late) in children with ears operated at 2–7 years of age compared with ears operated at 8–14 years of age

	2–7 years, %				8–14 years, %			
	absolute hearing		air-bone gap		absolute hearing		air-bone gap	
	0–20 dB	0–30 dB	0–10 dB	0–20 dB	0–20 dB	0–30 dB	0–10 dB	0–20 dB
Preoperatively	19	50	0	27	19	41	6	27
Primarily	65	88	58	81	65	87	46	81
Late	80	88	64	88	72	88	54	89

Preoperative and primarily numbers aged 2–7 are 26, late numbers are 25. Corresponding numbers aged 8–14 are 98 and 85 ears.

children, and in 89% of the elder children (table II). We did not find any difference in the hearing results, whether the operation was done on a moist ear, or whether it was done on dry ear. The best results were obtained in ears with an intact ossicular chain, and the poorest results were seen in ears which lacked the stapes arcade. There was one 'dead ear' following surgery in our series.

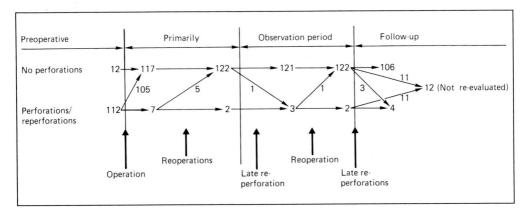

Fig. 1. The connections between perforations, reperforations, and graft-takes from the preoperative period, through the primary period (6 months to 2 years postoperatively) and the observation period, to the last follow-up. There were 7 primary perforations (within the first 2 postoperative years), and 4 secondary perforations.

Tympanometry

Tympanometry was performed in 110 ears, of which 70% showed a tympanogramme type A (+99 to −99 mm H_2O), 14% type C_1 (−100 to −199 mm H_2O), 6% type C_2 (−200 to −399 mm H_2O), and 6% type B (−400 mm H_2O or less). Four percent had perforations of the tympanic membrane. The tensa was adherent and retracted in 5 ears, retracted without adhesion in 3 ears, and rigid in 4 ears.

Cholesteatomas

During the observation period one ear was reoperated because of cholesteatoma. At the follow-up we found cholesteatoma in one ear. Both cholesteatomas were attic cholesteatomas.

Discussion and Conclusion

With a graft-take rate of 92%, and with only 4 ears developing late perforation (we have an observation time up to 15 years), and with no more perforations in the younger children than in the elder children, we share the opinion of Smyth and Hassard [2], and of Armstrong and Char-

lotte [7], that tympanoplasty can be done at any age. Age per se is no
contraindication for operation. All our operations were one-stage procedures, and the results compared to the results obtained by two-stage procedures, do not in our opinion indicate the necessity of staging the operation [3, 8]. Postoperative, secretory otitis was no problem in our patients.
Only 5% needed insertion of a grommet during the observation period.
Only 12% had tympanogrammes type B or C_2, mostly because of adhesions retractions or rigid tympanic membranes. Further and more-detailed
results have been published elsewhere [9]. During the observation period
attic cholesteatomas developed in 2 ears, there were no tensa cholesteatomas, and the tympanoplasties can perhaps be the reason, if retraction of
the Shrapnell membrane is due to negative pressure of the middle ear after
closing of the perforation. There were no signs of cholesteatomas developing directly from the tympanoplasty. Cholesteatomas were not included in
this series, but late results of treatment of cholesteatomas have been analyzed by the authors [10].

We have in our series 69% with an intact ossicular chain, which is
much higher than in adults [11, 12]. An early operation may prevent progression of ossicular chain pathology.

The hearing results are as good in children as in adults, and the late
results are even better. It is well known that late hearing results decline by
increasing observation time in adults [12].

The indications for tympanoplasty in children may be wide: hearing
loss, bilateral perforations, great desire for bathing or swimming, recurrent
discharge. If possible, the ear should be dry at the time of operation, but
even when the ear has not become dry by conservative treatment, surgery
can be performed anyway, as the results are as good as in dry ears.

No recurrent upper respiratory infections should be present, when you
perform the tympanoplasty.

References

1   Bluestone, C.D.; Cantekin, E.I.; Douglas, G.S.: Eustachian tube function related to
    the results of tympanoplasty in children. Laryngoscope *89:* 1–9 (1979).
2   Smyth, G.D.L.; Hassard, T.H.: Tympanoplasty in children. Am. J. Otol. *1:* 199–205
    (1980).
3   Gans, H.: Tympanoplasty in children. Archs Otolar. *77:* 350–352 (1963).
4   Kleinfeldt, D.; Vick, U.; Hoffmann, M.: Probleme und Ergebnisse der Tympano-
    plastiken im Kindesalter. Dt. Gesundh-Wes. *25:* 2338–2342 (1970).

5 Buchwald, K.A.; Birck, H.: Serous otitis media and type I tympanoplasty in children. Ann. Otol. Rhinol. Lar. *89:* suppl. 68, pp. 324–325 (1980).
6 Raine, C.H.; Singh, S.D.: Tympanoplasty in children. A review of 114 cases. J. Lar. Otol. *97:* 217–221 (1983).
7 Armstrong, B.W.; Charlotte, N.C.: Tympanoplasty in children. Laryngoscope *75:* 1062–1069 (1965).
8 Palva, T.; Holopainen, E.: Management of noncholesteatomatous suppurative middle ear disease in children. Adv. Otorhinolar. *23:* 45–57 (1978).
9 Lau, T.; Tos, M.: Tympanoplasty in children. An analysis of late results. Am. J. Otol. *7:* 55–59 (1986).
10 Lau, T.; Tos, M.: Cholesteatoma in children. Recurrence related to observation period. Am. J. Otolar. (in press, 1987).
11 Tos, M.: Pathology of the ossicular chain in various chronic middle ear diseases. J. Lar. Otol. *93:* 769–780 (1979).
12 Tos, M.: Tympanoplasty results and age. Archs Otolar. *96:* 493–498 (1972).

Torben Lau, MD, ENT Department, Gentofte University Hospital,
DK–2900 Hellerup (Denmark)

Subject Index

THE MANCHESTER MEDICAL SOCIETY

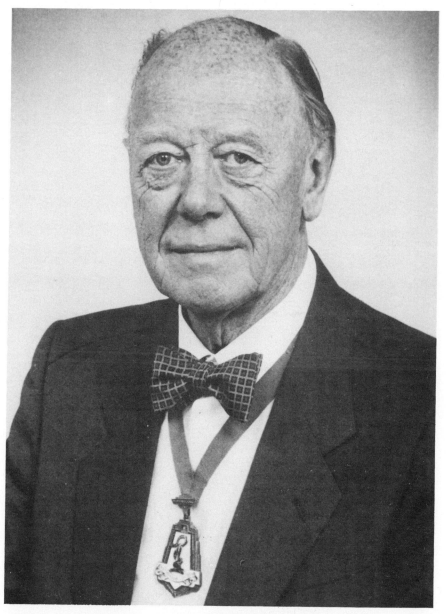

Professor J C Brocklehurst CBE, MD, FRCP
President 1990-91

ANNUAL REPORT

OF THE

MANCHESTER

MEDICAL SOCIETY

1989-90

CONTENTS

**Will Fellows, Members and Associates please inform
the Administrator when they change their post,
address or gain additional qualifications**

Manchester Medical Society

MANCHESTER MEDICAL SOCIETY

PROVISIONAL PROGRAMME
FOR THE SESSION 1990/91

1990
OCTOBER

Wednesday 3rd, 2 pm
Joint Meeting the Department of Cardiology, Wythenshawe Hospital (at Wythenshawe)
Pharmax Cardiovascular Exchange

(Medicine)
Cardiology Symposium

Wednesday 3rd, 5.15 pm (at Wythenshawe)
Presidential Address
Dr C BRAY

(Medicine)
Treatment of myocardial infarction around the world

Tuesday 9th, 8 pm
Presidential Address
Mr R J BARNARD

(Surgery)

Urological salvage

Wednesday 10th, 5.30 pm
Dr A J HOWAT

(Pathology)
Nucleolar organiser regions in histopathology

Thursday 11th, 8.15 pm
Presidential Address
Dr J M ANDERTON

(Anaesthesia)

"Doctor, I feel faint"

Thursday 18th, 6 pm
Dr ANTOINETTE CHALLEN

(Paediatrics)
Diabetes and family stress

Tuesday 23rd, 5.30 pm
Professor W I FRASER

(Psychiatry)
Aspects of language for psychiatrists

Wednesday 24th, 5.30 pm
Professor J C BROCKLEHURST

(Society)
Aging - yesterday, today and tomorrow

Thursday 25th, 5.30 pm
Professor S P B DONNAN

(Public Health Medicine)

Monday 29th, 6 pm
Presidential Address
Mr P R WHITE

(Odontology)

Dentogeneology

NOVEMBER

Wednesday 7th, 5.30 pm
Joint Meeting with North West Regional Association of Physicians (at North Manchester)
Professor M B PEPYS

(Medicine)

New images of clinical amyloidosis

Thursday 13th, 8 pm
Mr R S SNEATH

(Surgery)
Orthopaedic oncology

2

Wednesday 14th, 5.30pm Dr D W DAWSON	(Pathology) Cobalamin deficiency
Thursday 22nd, 5.30 pm Professor R E Klein	(Public Health Medicine) An outsider's view of the NHS Review
Thursday 22nd, 8.15 pm Dr A I J Brain	(Anaesthesia) Experience with laryngeal mask airway
Monday 26th, 6 pm Mr H S ORTON	(Odontology) Functional appliances in orthodontic treatment - what they are and how they work
Tuesday 27th, 5.30 pm Professor G EDWARDS	(Psychiatry) Recovery from alcoholism

DECEMBER

Tuesday 11th, 5.30 pm Professor G D CHISHOLM	(Surgery) Dilemmas and decisions in prostate cancer
Wednesday 12th, 2 pm Christmas Lecture for Young People Mr J F DARK	(Society) Heart surgery - what it is and how it developed
Wednesday 12th, 5.30 pm Dr A D H WYLLIE	(Pathology) Genetic mechanisms in cancer
Thursday 13th, 6 pm Presidential Address Dr J L Burn	(Paediatrics) "Feed my lambs... tend my sheep" - the sanctity of family care
Thursday 13th, 8.15 pm Dr N M DEARDEN	(Anaesthesia) Aspects of neuro-anaesthesia

1991
JANUARY

Tuesday 8th, 8 pm Mr M MUGHAL	(Surgery) Minimally invasive surgery - fact or fantasy
Wednesday 9th, 5.30pm Professor J P BURNIE	(Pathology) Heat shock proteins and fungi
Thursday 17th, 8.15 pm Professor I ISHERWOOD	(Anaesthesia) Imaging in the future
Tuesday 22nd, 5.30 pm Dr B LASK	(Psychiatry) Somatization in children
Thursday 24th, 5.30 pm Ms SARAH PARKIN	(Public Health Medicine) Green and public health
Monday 28th, 6pm Alan Hilton Medal & Members' Evening	(Odontology)

FEBRUARY

Tuesday 12th, 8 pm   (Surgery)
Michael Boyd Memorial Lecture
Professor I E GILLESPIE   The rise and fall of gastric surgery

Wednesday 13th, 5.30 pm   (Medicine & Pathology)
Dr J A KANIS   Therapeutic modulation of bone remodelling
                                                        with diphosphonates

Thursday 14th, 8.15 pm   (Anaesthesia)
Papers for the ICI and Abbott Registrars' Prizes and AGM

Wednesday 20th, 10.30 am.   Society
Full Day Symposim   Quality and Outcome of medical care

Wednesday 20th, 5.30 pm   (Society)
Telford Memorial Lecture   Genetics and the human race - disaster or
Dr BERNADETTE MODELL   salvation?

Thursday 21st, 6 pm   (Paediatrics)
Dr J M COURIEL   Paediatric support after sudden infant death

Monday 25th, 6 pm   (Odontology)
Mr R J WILLIAMS   Surgical aspects of parotid gland disease

Tuesday 26th, 5.30 pm   (Psychiatry)
Professor J F W DEAKIN   Brain mechanisms in the social origin of
                                                        affective disorders

Thursday 28th, 5.30 pm   (Public Health Medicine)
Students' Presentations of Work in Public Health

MARCH

Wednesday 6th, 10.00 am   (Medicine)
Joint Meeting with the Department of Gastroenterology, Victoria Hospital (in Blackpool)
Symposium (in Blackpool)   Gastroenterology

Thursday 7th, 6 pm   (Society)
Joint Meeting with the Liverpool Medical Institution (in Manchester)
Dr R M PHILPOTT   New directions in long-term psychogeriatric care
Dr S SALTISSI   Modern thinking on ischaemic heart disease

Tuesday 12th, 8 pm   (Surgery)
Papers for the ICI Surgical Registrars' Evening

Wednesday 13th, 5.30 pm   (Pathology)
Trainees' Evening

Friday 15th, 8.15 pm   (Anaesthesia)
Joint Meeting with the Liverpool Society of Anaesthetists (in Liverpool)
Dr Eleanor VIVORI   Head injuries
Dr S G GREENHOUGH   Fibreoptic intubation in paediatric practice

4

Thursday 21st, 5.30 pm
Professor ELAINE MURPHY
(Public Health Medicine)
Whither community care?

Monday 25th, 6 pm
Dr D G MACDONALD
(Odontology)
Whose teeth - Forensic Odontology

Tuesday 26th, 5.30 pm
Professor P J HUXLEY
(Psychiatry)
Beyond the cardboard box: continuing crises in the social care of mental illness

APRIL

Wednesday 3rd, 6 pm
Prize Evening
(Medicine)

Monday 8th, 5.30 pm
British Lung Foundation Lecture
Sir Richard DOLL, FRS
(Society)
Smoking and lung disease, 40 years on

Tuesday 9th, 8 pm
Symposium
(Surgery)
Imaging techniques

Wednesday 10th, 5.30 pm
Presidential Address
Dr K P SITLANI
(Pathology)
Twenty one years on

Thursday 11th, 6 pm
Symposium
(Paediatrics)
Recent advances in cystic fribosis

Thursday 11th, 8.15 pm
Out of Town Meeting (in Blackpool)
Symposium
(Anaesthesia)
Blood and the anaesthetist

Tuesday 23rd, 5.30 pm
Presidential Address
Dr S BENJAMIN
(Psychiatry)
Chronic pain and illness behaviour

Thursday 25th, 5.30 pm
Presidential Address
Professor I LECK
(Public Health Medicine)

Monday 29th, 6 pm
Professor R M BASKER
(Odontology)
The denture collector

MAY

Wednesday 1st, 5.30 pm
Annual General Meeting
(Society)

Thursday 9th, 8.15 pm
ICI Anaesthesia Manchester Medal Inaugural Lecture (at Alderley Park)
Dr M W JOHNSTONE
(Anaesthesia)
Fifty years in Anaesthesia

5

Honorary Fellows

Professor Sir DOUGLAS BLACK, MD, FRCP
DAVID FREDERICK COOK, MA, DipArchAdmin, DipLib
Professor Sir W MANSFIELD COOPER, LLM
DAVID LLOYD GRIFFITHS, FRCS
ANDREW RENNIE HUNTER, MD, MB, ChB, FRFPS, FRCS, FFARCS, DA
Dame HILDA NORA LLOYD, DBE, FRCS, FRCOG
JOHN FREDERICK WILKINSON, MD, MSc, PhD, FRCP, DSc, FRSC

Honorary Members

Section of Pathology

PETER MAXWELL FARROW BISHOP, DM, FRCP
CECIL GEORGE PAINE, MD, FRCOG

Section of Anaesthesia

ANDREW RENNIE HUNTER, MD, MB, ChB, FRFPS, FRCS, FFARCS, DA
MICHAEL WILLIAM JOHNSTONE, MB, BCh, BAO, FFARCS, DA, RCPSI
FRANK LEONARD ROBERTSHAW, MB, ChB, FFARCS, DA, DObstRCOG

Section of Odontology

COLIN COOKE, LDS, FDSRCS
PAMELA HOBSON, MSc, LDS, DDS
JAMES KENNETH HOLT, MSc, LDS, DDS, FDSRCS
JOHN HAMILTON HOWARTH, LDS, BDS
ALAN WELDON MOULE, LDS, BDS, FDSRCS
JOAN EDITH STONER, BDS

Past Presidents of the Society

The names of those deceased are printed in italics.

Elected

SEPTEMBER,	1834	*JOHN HULL, MD*
OCTOBER,	1838	*JAMES LOMAX BARDSLEY, MD*
„	1843	*WILLIAM JAMES WILSON, FRCS*
„	1845	*JAMES LOMAX BARDSLEY, MD*
„	1848	*THOMAS RADFORD, MD*
„	1849	*THOMAS ASHTON, MD*

Office of President abolished Oct., 1850; the Treasurer of the Society to be ex officio Chairman of its Meetings

OCT. 1850 to DEC. 1858

TREASURER: *JOHN WINDSOR, FRCS*

Office of President re-established January, 1859

JANUARY,	1859	*JOHN WINDSOR, FRCS*
„	1860	*SAMUEL CROMPTON, MRCS*
„	1861	*CHARLES CLAY, LRCS (Edin.)*
„	1862	*LOUIS BORCHARDT, MD*
„	1863	*EDWARD LUND, FRCS*
„	1864	*DANIEL NOBLE, MD*
„	1865	*WILLIAM ROBERTS, MD*
„	1866	*THOMAS WINDSOR, MRCS*
„	1867	*HENRY BROWNE, MD*
„	1868	*THOMAS MELLOR, FRCS*
„	1869	*HENRY SIMPSON, MD*
„	1870	*JAMES OGDEN FLETCHER, MD*
„	1871	*JOHN THORBURN, MD*
„	1872	*JOHN GALT, FRCS*
„	1873	*DAVID LLOYD ROBERTS, MD, MRCP*
„	1874	*JOHN EDWARD MORGAN, MD, FRCP*
„	1876	*ARTHUR RANSOME, MD*
„	1878	*FREDERICK ASHTON HEATH, MRCS*
„	1880	*DAVID LITTLE, MD*
„	1881	*EDWARD LUND, FRCS*
„	1883	*DANIEL JOHN LEECH, MD, FRCP*
„	1885	*WALTER WHITEHEAD, FRCS (Edin.)*
„	1886	*JAMES HARDIE, FRCS*
„	1888	*JULIUS DRESCHFELD, MD, FRCP*
„	1889	*JAMES ROSS, MD, FRCP*
„	1891	*THOMAS JONES, BS, FRCS*
„	1892	*ALFRED WILLIAM STOCKS, MRCS*
„	1893	*CHARLES EDWARD GLASCOTT, MD*
„	1894	*JOHN DIXON MANN, MD, FRCP*
„	1895	*FREDERICK ARMITAGE SOUTHAM, FRCS*
„	1896	*HENRY ASHBY, MD, FRCP*
„	1897	*GRAHAM STEELL, MD, FRCP*
„	1898	*GEORGE ARTHUR WRIGHT, MB, FRCS*
„	1899	*WILLIAM JAPP SINCLAIR, MD, MRCP*
„	1900	*THOMAS CARLTON RAILTON, MD, MRCP*
„	1901	*ALFRED HARRY YOUNG, MB, FRCS*
„	1902	*THOMAS HARRIS, MD, FRCP*
„	1903	*ABRAHAM MATTHEWSON EDGE, MD*
„	1904	*JUDSON SYKES BURY, MD, FRCP*
„	1905	*WILLIAM THORBURN, FRCS*

```
JANUARY,  1906    SAMUEL BUCKLEY, MD
    ”     1907    SIEGMUND MORITZ, MD, MRCP
    ”     1908    ARTHUR THOMAS WILKINSON, MD, FRCP
    ”     1909    Sir WILLIAM COATES, CB, LRCP, MRCS
    ”     1910    EDWARD STANMORE BISHOP, FRCS
    ”     1911    ABRAHAM EMRYS JONES, MD
    ”     1912    ERNEST SEPTIMUS REYNOLDS, MD, FRCP
    ”     1913    JOSHUA JOHN COX, MD
    ”     1914–18  ARCHIBALD DONALD, MD, FRCP
    ”     1919    JOHN WILLIAM SMITH, FRCS
    ”     1920    ROBERT BRIGGS WILD, MD, FRCP
    ”     1921    THOMAS ASHTON GOODFELLOW, CBE, MD
    ”     1922–23  Sir WILLIAM MILLIGAN, MD
  MAY,    1923–24  EDWARD MANSFIELD BROCKBANK, MBE, MD, FRCP
    ”     1924–25  GEORGE REDMAYNE MURRAY, MD, FRCP, DCL
    ”     1925–26  ARTHUR HENRY BURGESS, MSc, FRCS
    ”     1926–27  ALFRED ALEXANDER MUMFORD, BSc, MD
    ”     1927–28  JOHN GRAY CLEGG, MD, BS, FRCS
    ”     1928–29  RICHARD WALTER MARSDEN, BSc, MD, MRCP
    ”     1929–30  ALBERT RAMSBOTTOM, MC, MD, FRCP
    ”     1930–31  JOHN HOWSON RAY, ChM, FRCS
    ”     1931–32  JOHN SEBASTIAN BACH STOPFORD, MBE, MD, FRS
    ”     1932–33  EVELYN DAVISON TELFORD, MA, MSc, FRCS
    ”     1933–34  CHARLES PAGET LAPAGE, MD, FRCP
    ”     1934–35  ERNEST BOSDIN LEECH, MA, MD, FRCP
    ”     1935–36  ARNOLD GREGORY, MRCS, LRCP
    ”     1936–37  GARNETT WRIGHT, FRCS
    ”     1937–38  WILLIAM FLETCHER SHAW, MD, FRCP, FRCOG
    ”     1938–39  HENRY STANLEY RAPER, CBE, MD, DSc, FRS
    ”     1939–43  THOMAS HERBERT OLIVER, MA, MD, FRCP
    ”     1943–44  CATHERINE CHISHOLM, CBE, BA, MD
    ”     1944–45  FREDERIC WOOD JONES, MB, DSc, FRCS, FRS
    ”     1945–46  WILSON HAROLD HEY, FRCS
    ”     1946–47  DANIEL DOUGAL, MC, MD, FRCOG
    ”     1947–48  JOHN MORLEY, ChM, FRCS
    ”     1948–49  GEOFFREY JEFFERSON, MS, FRCS, FRS
    ”     1949–50  ARTHUR HILLYARD HOLMES, MD, FRCP

              The Society was reconstituted in 1950
_____

    ”     1950–51  WILSON HAROLD HEY, FRCS
    ”     1951–52  Sir WILLIAM FLETCHER SHAW, MD, FRCP, FRCOG
    ”     1952–53  JOHN CRIGHTON BRAMWELL, MA, MD, FRCP
    ”     1953–54  JOHN MORLEY, ChM, FRCS
    ”     1954–55  HUGH PATRICK FAY, MB, ChB
    ”     1955–56  WILLIAM BROCKBANK, MD, FRCP
    ”     1956–57  JOHN FREDERICK WILKINSON, MD, MSc, DSc, PhD, FRCP, FRSC
    ”     1957–58  ROBERT LEECH NEWELL, MD, FRCS, LRCP
    ”     1958–59  FERGUS ROBERT FERGUSON, MD, FRCP
    ”     1959–60  CHARLES ERNEST SYKES, TD, FFA, RCS
    ”     1960–61  WALTER SCHLAPP, MB, ChB, MSc, PhD
    ”     1961–62  HARRY TEESDALE SIMMONS, MD, FRCS
    ”     1962–63  Lord PLATT, MSc, MD, FRCP
    ”     1963–64  VICTOR FRANCIS LAMBERT, MD, FRCS, ChM
    ”     1964–65  GEORGE ARCHIBALD GRANT MITCHELL, OBE, TD, MB, ChM, DSc
    ”     1965–66  ERIC DUFF GREY, MA, MD, DMRE, FFR
    ”     1966–67  RONALD EPEY LANE, CBE, MD, FRCP
```

MAY,	1967-68	DENIS SMITH POOLE-WILSON, BA, MCh, FRCS, FRCSI
"	1968-69	*ALAN HOWARD HILTON, LDS, FLS*
"	1969-70	*ARTHUR MORGAN JONES, MSc, FRCP*
"	1970-71	ALEXANDER COLIN PATTON CAMPBELL, MSc. FRCP, FRCPath
"	1971-72	WILLIAM FRANCIS NICHOLSON, MBE, MA, MD, FRCS
"	1972-73	*MARTIN CYRIL GORDON ISRAELS, MSc, MD, FRCP*
"	1973-74	*ARON HOLZEL, MD, FRCP*
"	1974-75	THOMAS MOORE, MD, FRCP
"	1975-76	HENRY TAYLOR HOWAT, CBE, MD, FRCP
"	1976-77	*PATRICK SARSFIELD BYRNE, CBE, MSC, FRCGP*
"	1977-78	AMBROSE JOLLEYS, MD, FRCS
"	1978-79	ANDREW RENNIE HUNTER, MD, DA, FFARCS, FRFPS, FRCS
"	1979-80	SAMUEL OLEESKY, FRCP, MD
"	1980-81	ALAN HADFIELD GOWENLOCK, MSC, PhD, FRCPath, FRCS
"	1981-82	NORTHAGE JOHN DE VILLE MATHER, MA, MB, ChB, DPM, FRCPsych
"	1982-83	JOSEPH REGINALD MOORE, OBE, MDS, MSc, FDSRCS
"	1983-84	RHYS TUDOR WILLIAMS, MB, BChir, FRCP
"	1984-85	SYDNEY WILLIAM STANBURY, MD, MB, ChB, FRCP
"	1985-86	IAN ISHERWOOD, MD, FRCP, FRCR, FFR, RCSI(Hon)
"	1986-87	RICHARD WAYWELL BURSLEM, MD, FRCOG
"	1987-88	ERNEST ALWYN SMITH, CBE, MB, ChB, PhD, MSc, DPH, FRCP, FFCM, RFCGP
"	1988-89	CLIFFORD RALPH KAY, CBE, MD, PhD, FRCGP
"	1989-90	JOHN FAIRMAN DARK, BSc, MB, ChB, FRCS

Past Hon. Secretaries

1834–35	JOHN WALKER, LFP and S
1834–38	JOSEPH PEEL CATLOW, MRCS
1835–38	PHILIP HENRY HOLLAND, MRCS
1838–39	DANIEL NOBLE, MD
1838–40	JOHN WALKER, LFP and S
1840–41	HENRY W KER, MRCS
1840–43	MICHAEL SATTERTHWAITE, MD
1841–43	THOMAS FREDERICK BROWNBILL, FRCS
1843–44	SAMUEL CROMPTON, MRCS
1843–45	THOMAS DORRINGTON, MRCS
1844–46	ISAAC A FRANKLIN, MRCS
1845–50	FRANK RENAUD, MD
1846–50	HENRY REID, MD
1850–53	EDWARD LUND, MRCS
1853–56	RALPH WORTHINGTON LEDWARD, MRCS
1856–58	SAMUEL CROMPTON, MRCS
1859	THOMAS WINDSOR, MRCS
1859–63	WILLIAM ROBERTS, MD
1864–67	JOHN THORBURN, MD
1868–71	WILLIAM HEATH, MRCS
1872–73	CHRISTOPHER CURRIE RITCHIE, MD
1874–78	WALTER WHITEHEAD, LSA, FRCS (Edin.)
1879–84	CHARLES JAMES CULLINGWORTH, MRCS, MRCP
1885–89	FREDERICK ARMITAGE SOUTHAM, FRCS
1890–93	THOMAS CARLETON RAILTON, MD, MRCP
1894–98	WILLIAM COATES, CB, LRCP, MRCS
1899–1901	ERNEST SEPTIMUS REYNOLDS, MD, FRCP
1902–05	JOHN EDWARD PLATT, FRCS
1906–07	RICHARD WALTER MARSDEN, MD, MRCP
1908–10	EVELYN DAVISON TELFORD, FRCS
1911–18	ERNEST BOSDIN LEECH, MD (assisted by CHARLES POWELL WHITE, MD, FRCS)
1919–20	WILSON HAROLD HEY, FRCS
1920–24	ROBERT GIBSON, MD
1924–26	ARTHUR HILLYARD HOLMES, MD, FRCP
1926–28	JOHN CRIGHTON BRAMWELL, MD, FRCP
1928–30	ALEXANDER GRAHAM BRYCE, MD, FRCS
1930–32	FERGUS ROBERT FERGUSON, MD, FRCP
1932–34	DONALD McKAY SUTHERLAND, MD, FRCS
1934–36	WILLIAM BROCKBANK, MD, FRCP
1936–47	REGINALD ELLIS, MD, FRCP
1947–49	GEORGE GEOFFREY EVANSON SMYTH, MD, FRCP
1949–50	HENRY TAYLOR HOWAT, FRCP, FRCPE

1950–54	WILLIAM BROCKBANK, MD, FRCP
1954–57	HENRY TAYLOR HOWAT, FRCP, FRCPE
1957–59	DOUGLAS ANDREW KILGOUR BLACK, MD, FRCP
1959–63	EDWARD GEOFFREY WADE, MD, FRCP
1963–66	SAMUEL OLEESKY, MSc, MD, FRCP
1966–70	GEOFFREY HOWITT, MD, FRCP
1970–74	HAROLD FRANK McGHIE BASSETT, FRCS
1974–78	DONALD GRAHAM DUNLOP DAVIDSON, FFARCS
1978–85	WILLIS JOHN ELWOOD, MB, BCh, BAO, FFCM, DPH
1985–88	BARRY ANTHONY ENOCH, MB, ChB, FRCP

Past Hon. Treasurers

1834–41	THOMAS RADFORD, MD
1841–42	SAMUEL BARTON, FRCS
1842–49	THOMAS ASHTON, MD
1849–58	JOHN WINDSOR, FRCS
1859	DANIEL NOBLE, MD
1860–62	JOHN WINDSOR, FRCS
1863–65	LOUIS BORCHARDT, MD
1866–72	EDWARD LUND, MRCS
1873–78	JOHN THORBURN, MD
1879	DAVID LITTLE, MD
1880–81	FREDERICK ASHTON HEATH, MRCS
1882–86	DAVID LITTLE, MD
1887–1900	CHARLES EDWARD GLASCOTT, MD
1901–07	JOHN WILLIAM SMITH, FRCS
1908	SIMEON HOLGATE OWEN, MD
1909–18	RICHARD WALTER MARSDEN, MD, MRCP
1919–25	FRANK EDWARD TYLECOTE, MD, FRCP
1925–30	JOHN FORBES WARD, MD, MRCP
1930–35	EDWARD STANLEY BRENTNALL, FRCS (Edin.)
1935–39	ALEXANDER ROBERT SOMERFORD, MD
1939–46	REGINALD ELLIS, MD, FRCP
1946–50	ALEX LOMAX KENYON, FRCS

1950–52	JAMES KENNETH HOLT, MSc, FDSRCS, DDS
1952–57	CHARLES ERNEST SYKES, DA, FFA, RCS
1957–65	ANDREW RENNIE HUNTER, MD, DA, FFARCS, FRFPS, FRCS
1965–69	ANTHONY REX ANSCOMBE, FRCS
1969–73	ALAN HADFIELD GOWENLOCK, MSc, PhD, FRCPath, FRSC
1973–76	JOHN TERENCE PATTON, RD, FRCR
1976–85	JOHN GRAHAM BUCHANAN RUSSELL, MB, ChB, FRCR, FFR, DMRD, DCH, DObst, RCOG
1985–88	WILLIS JOHN ELWOOD, MB, BCh, BAO, FFCM, DPH

Telford Memorial Lectures

1964-65	Sir JAMES LEARMOUTH	Surgery in a developing society
1965-66	Dr F H C CRICK	The genetic code
1966-67	Dr RICHARD DOLL	The geographical distribution of cancer
1967-68	Professor E B CHAIN	Biochemical research and progress in medicine
1968-69	Professor J Z YOUNG	Logic and language in relation to brain structure
1970-71	Sir SOLLY ZUCKERMAN	Two Manchester anatomists
1971-72	Sir DERRICK DUNLOP	The problem of modern medicines and their control
1972-73	Hon Sir JOSEPH CANTLEY	Treatment of the offender
1973-74	Professor DOROTHY HODGKIN	Insulin
1974-75	Dr H YELLOWLEES	To promote the establishment of a comprehensive health service
1975-76	Dr R Y CALNE	The current state of organ transplantation
1976-77	Professor W S PEART	The kidney as an endocrine organ
1977-78	Sir RODNEY SMITH	The patient with cancer and his doctor
1978-79	Sir DOUGLAS BLACK	Medicine and Society
1979-80	Sir ALEC MERRISON	Patient and provider: the idea of a health service
1980-81	Professor ALAN EMERY	Medical genetics-the preventive medicine of the future
1981-82	Professor JOHN A DAVIS	The past, present and future of neonatology
1982-83	Professor Sir WILLIAM TRETHOWAN, OBE	Growing old gracefully
1983-84	Professor J B WEST	Human physiology on the summit of Mount Everest
1984-85	Professor Sir FRED HOYLE	Life as a cosmic phenomenon
1985-86	Dr E D ACHESON	Public Health - yesterday, today and tomorrow
1986-87	Sir CYRIL CLARKE, KBE	Longevity: nurture versus nature
1987-88	Professor J M BLISS	The discovery of insulin
1988-89	Professor Sir GEOFFREY SLANEY, KBE	Six centuries of surgeons
1989-90	Lord WALTON OF DETCHANT	Professional responsibility

Christmas Lectures for Young People

1975-76	Dr S OLEESKY	Medicine and history
1976-77	Professor I ISHERWOOD	Radiology in history and antiquity
1977-78	Dr G W BOWEN Dr J C FRANKLAND	Medicine on the highest and lowest planes-the story of mountain and cave rescue
1978-79	Professor I E GILLESPIE	Decisions, decisions
1979-80	Professor E A SMITH	What can we do about cancer?
1980-81	Dr M LONGSON	Viruses and man-a cloak and dagger story?
1981-82	Professor I ISHERWOOD	Twentieth-century man-the inside story
1982-83	Professor R M CASE	Disease: lessons for science and society
1983-84	Professor R HARRIS	Genes and the future of medicine
1984-85	Professor M IRVING	Coping with catastrophe
1985-86	Dr D ROWLANDS	Heart disease-the modern plague
1986-87	Dr E TAPP Mr R NEAVE	Heads and Tales
1987-88	Dr D DONNAI	Myths and malformations
1988-89	Professor W I N KESSEL	Madmen and geniuses
1989-90	Dr J B GARLAND	The Grand Duke and after: Manchester, medicine and industry in the 19th century

Honorary Secretary's Report
for the Session 1989-90

Since its re-formation in 1950 the tradition of the Society has been to hold a number of meetings in addition to those organised by the individual sections. This year there were six such meetings all followed by an informal dinner in the University Refectory at which the speakers were the guests of honour.

The session commenced with the Presidential Address by Mr John F Dark on Wednesday 25th October 1989. Before his retirement Mr Dark was Consultant Thoracic Surgeon for the Manchester Area Health Authority and appropriately his address was entitled "Thoracoplasty to heart transplant: forty years in the chest". His vivid account of his own work and that of his colleagues at Wythenshawe Hospital was greatly appreciated by an audience drawn from a wide range of disciplines. At this meeting Professor A R Hunter was elected as an Honorary Fellow of the Society in recognition of his long and loyal service. His service on the Council of the Society began in 1956 and since then he has held office as President (1978-79), Honorary Treasurer (1957-65), Trustee (1968-90) and Honorary Librarian (1976-78).

The next event in the Society's calendar was the Christmas Lecture for Young People which took place on Wednesday 13th December 1989. For a number of years the lecture had been over-subscribed and the Society had to look beyond the University's Medical School to find suitable accommodation. The venue chosen was the main lecture theatre of the Roscoe Building and some four hundred young people attended. The speaker was Dr John Garland (Consultant Urologist, North Manchester, Salford Royal and Royal Manchester Children's Hospitals) and his address was "The Grand Duke and after: Manchester, medicine and industry in the 19th Century". He gave a detailed and expert account of how the effects of Manchester's earlier industries had produced environmental and industrial diseases which still involve physicians and surgeons today.

The Society was delighted that Lord Walton of Detchant (former President of the General Medical Council and former Warden of Green College, Oxford) was able to accept the invitation to give the Telford Memorial Lecture. This was held on Wednesday 14th February 1990 and his very topical title was "Professional responsibility". The lecture, like so many of the Society's events, attracted both academic and hospital staff, all of whom appreciated Lord Walton's excellent address.

Unlike the Christmas Lecture, the joint meeting with the Liverpool Medical Institution, once the highlight of the Society's Annual programme, is now very poorly attended. Less than twenty people made the journey to Liverpool on Thursday 1st March 1990 to hear two excellent addresss and to enjoy the hospitality of the Institution at the dinner afterwards. The records of both organisations have details of the large number of members who used to attend the joint meetings. In those days travel was by train and, so popular were the events, a special train was sometimes hired for the occasion. The speakers this year were Mr David Gough (Consultant Paediatric Urologist, Royal Manchester Children's Hospital) whose title was "Congenital anomalies of the penis and their treatment" and Dr Colin Bray (Consultant Cardiologist, Wythenshawe Hospital and Manchester Royal Infirmary) who spoke on "Modern management of myocardial infarction".

The second British Lung Foundation Lecture hosted by the Society took place on Tuesday 3rd April 1990 and this year the lecturer was Professor Margaret Turner-Warwick (President of the Royal College of Physicians). Her title was "What is clinical research? Do we make the most of natural experiments?" The lecture, which was once again sponsored by Duncan Flockhart Limited, was extremely well received by a lively audience.

The Annual General Meeting took place on Wednesday 2nd May 1990 when Mr John Wallwork (Consultant Thoracic Surgeon, Papworth Hospital) gave an address entitled "Progress in heart-lung transplantation". His lively account of the work carried out in this field was an excellent finale to the 1989/90 programme.

The membership of the Society remains fairly constant and at the end of 1989 stood at 2120 as compared with 2149 at the end of 1988. The following table shows the breakdown of this total:

Honorary Fellows	7
Honorary Members of Sections (not being Honorary Fellows)	10
Life Fellows (not being Honorary Fellows or Honorary Members of Sections)	221
Fellows	1779
Temporary Members	19
Non-medical Associates	77
Members of Sections (not being Fellows)	7

At the beginning of 1990, having been Fellows for thirty-five years, the following were elected as Life Fellows: John Andrew Locke Cooper, John Wilkinson Ferguson, Philip William Gilman, Harold Hastings Gunson, Jean Millwood Halliwell, Charles Kirkham Heffernan, George Francis Wilkie Hossack, Gordon Daniel Jack, William Hugh Lyle, Eustace Peter Turner and Benjamin Newport White.

I regret to have to report the deaths of the following Life Fellows: Benjamin Leslie Alexander, Sylvia Kema Guthrie, James Ian Alexander Jamieson, George Marcus Komrower, Robert Michael Maher, Alfred William Lumsden Smith and George Geoffrey Smyth; and of Fellows; Ian Michael Brown, Andrew Maxwell Dickson, Syed Qamrul Hasan, Peter Ernest Penna and William Roy Swinburn.

This is my second report as Honorary Secretary of the Society and I cannot end it without thanking the staff of the Society, Mrs Barbara Lowndes, Administrator and her assistants Mrs Patricia Bowden and Miss Janet Hall for their help in keeping the Society running so smoothly. I know that their hard work is very much appreciated by all its members and particularly by the Honorary Officers of the Society and its Sections. It is with regret that I must report the resignation of Mrs Patricia Bowden who has been with the Society since September 1983. The Society extends its best wishes for her future happiness.

RORY FRANCIS McCLOY
Honorary Secretary

Honorary Treasurer's Report
for the Session 1989-90

During 1989, the second year of my term of office as Honorary Treasurer, the Society benefited from the increase in income consequent upon the rise in subscription rates which my predecessor advised. The number of fellows, members and associates having remained constant, there was a 25.2% increase in the subscription income received. The amount of money transferred from the Trustee's account was £25,200 which was 41% of the Society's expenditure. However, this includes the sum of £8,638 which was agreed for the purchase of new office equipment as well as a contribution to the general running costs of the Society.

On the expenditure side, the cost of employment of office and library staff increased by 9.4% as a result of incremental drift and salary inflation. As previously indicated, new equipment was purchased for the Society's office. The two items were a replacement photocopier and a new computer system. Both items should assist office efficiency and the latter item will provide the List of Fellows and aid preparation of the Annual Report. In the remainder of the non-staff costs, there has been a slight reduction in the expenditure in 1989 when compared with 1988. At the end of the year the Society's account showed a surplus of £1403.

I wish to express my thanks to the Society's staff Mrs Barbara Lowndes, Mrs Patricia Bowden and Miss Janet Hall for helping to contain office expenditure and for their general support during the year.

CAROLYN MARY JOHNSON
Honorary Treasurer

Trustee's Report
for the Session 1989-90

Despite the increased income which the Society is now receiving from subscriptions the transfer from the Trustees' Fund to the General Fund up to the end of 1989 amounted to approximately 40%. In fact the contribution from the Trustees increased from £20,500 in 1988 to £25,200 in 1989. This transfer has allowed the Society to make a substantial investment in new office equipment as well as meeting its general expenses.

In 1989 the income from the Trustees' investments, after allowing for income tax recovery, was almost £26,000 - a return of 6.2% on the market value of the total holdings which are about £416,000. During the year, on the advice of our stockbrokers, the Trustees altered some of their investments with the aim of increasing the annual income whilst still retaining an element of capital growth. By agreement with the Council of the Society, this policy will be continued for the immediate future.

As always, the Trustees' work has been made easier by the efficient book-keeping of Mrs Lowndes in the Society's office and by the advice of the Trustees' Department of of the National Westminster Bank plc and Bell Houldsworth Fairmont Limited, our stockbrokers.

Finally, the Trustees are delighted to record the award of the Honorary Fellowship of the Society to Professor A R Hunter, a Trustee since 1968.

ALAN HADFIELD GOWENLOCK
Trustee

INCOME AND EXPENDITURE ACCOUNT
FOR THE YEAR ENDED DECEMBER 31ST, 1989

	£	1989 £	£	1988 £
INCOME				
Subscriptions		34,936		27,894
Contribution re post graduate education		630		630
Bank interest received		447		250
Amount transferred from Trustees Account .		25,200		20,500
Other income		73		122
TOTAL INCOME FOR YEAR		£61,286		£49,396
EXPENDITURE				
Use of Library		500		500
Office Expenses:				
Clerical Assistance (including Pension Scheme)	23,801		20,563	
Printing and stationery	1,699		2,666	
Printing Annual Report	2,740		2,520	
Printing monthly diary	981		783	
Direct Debit Services	601		492	
Telephone	904		809	
Postages	2,792		2,715	
Sundries	345		291	
Repairs and renewals	1,637		1,803	
Purchase of new equipment and furniture	8,638		2,176	
		43,418		34,818
Meeting expenses:				
Meeting and lecturers' expenses	3,920		4,490	
Fee to Telford Lecturer	250		250	
Hire of rooms and projectionists' fee	507		416	
Refreshments	380		375	
		5,057		5,531
Grant to Library		9,089		8,855
Sundries:				
Accountancy and audit	1,639		1,495	
Accountancy (additional services)	-		230	
Bank Charges	100		75	
Gratuities	80		90	
Underprovision in previous year	-		150	
		1,819		2,040
TOTAL EXPENDITURE FOR THE YEAR		£59,883		£51,744
SURPLUS/(DEFICIT) FOR THE YEAR		£1,403		(£2,348)

BALANCE SHEET (GENERAL FUND) DECEMBER 31ST, 1989

	1989 £	1988 £
CURRENT LIABILITIES		
Creditors and accrued expenses	18,315	19,427
Amounts paid in advance	55	155
Pathology Trainees' Prizes	350	425
	18,720	20,007
CURRENT ASSETS		
Stocks of items for re-sale	3,438	3,630
Stationery stock	1,083	1,433
Debtors and prepaid expenses	1,005	1,593
Cash at bank	4,129	2,962
Cash in hand	79	-
	9,734	9,618
NET CURRENT LIABILITIES	(£8,986)	(£10,389)
Represented by:		
ACCUMULATED FUND		
Adverse balance 1st January, 1989	(10,389)	(8,041)
Surplus/(Deficit) for the year	1,403	(2,348)
Adverse balance 31st December, 1989	£8,986)	(£10,389)

BALANCE SHEET (TRUSTEES FUND) DECEMBER 31ST, 1989

	£	1989 £	£	1988 £
INVESTMENTS PER SCHEDULE at cost		235,713		188,834
(market value £415,838 - 1988 £347,866)				
INCOME TAX RECOVERABLE		6,468		5,648
DEBTOR				
Michael Boyd Memorial Lecture Fund ...		100		294
CASH AT BANK				
Capital account	4,424		403	
Income Account	2,889		2,552	
		7,313		2,955
		249,594		197,731
DUE TO KENNETH BLOOR TRAVELLING				
SCHOLARSHIP FUND		100		-
DUE TO MICHAEL BOYD MEMORIAL				
LECTURER		-		100
		£249,494		£197,631
Represented by:				
ACCUMULATED FUND				
Balance 1st January, 1989		197,631		190,976
Add:				
Income from investments	25,874		22,156	
Bank interest received	754		196	
Profit on sale of investments	50,702		5,123	
		77,330		27,475
		274,961		218,451
Deduct:				
Bank charges and expenses	267		320	
Transfer to general account	25,200		20,500	
		25,467		20,820
BALANCE 31ST DECEMBER 1989		£249,494		£197,631

MICHAEL BOYD MEMORIAL LECTURE FUND
BALANCE SHEET DECEMBER 31ST, 1989

	£	1989 £	£	1988 £
INVESTMENTS at cost		960		960
(£951 Treasury 8 3/4% loan 1997)				
(market value £867 - 1988 £877)				
INCOME TAX RECOVERABLE		21		22
CASH AT BANK				
Capital account	1		1	
Income account	185		395	
		186		396
		1,167		1,378
DUE TO TRUSTEES FUND		100		294
		£1,067		£1,084
Represented by:				
ACCUMULATED FUND				
Balance 1st January, 1989		1,084		1,101
Add:				
Investment income		83		83
		1,167		1,184
Memorial Lecturer's Fee		100		100
BALANCE 31ST DECEMBER 1989		£1,067		£1,084

KENNETH BLOOR TRAVELLING SCHOLARSHIP FUND
BALANCE SHEET DECEMBER 31ST, 1989

	£	1989 £	£	1988 £
INCOME TAX RECOVERABLE		465		293
CASH AT BANK		2,793		2,070
		3,258		2,363
OVERPAYMENT ON DEED OF COVENANT . .		-		(10)
DUE FROM TRUSTEES FUND		100		-
		£3,358		£2,353
Represented by:				
ACCUMULATED FUND				
Balance 1st January, 1989		2,353		588
Add:				
Donations by Deed of Covenant (Gross)	687		690	
Other Donations	180		1,035	
Bank interest received	138		40	
		1,005		1,765
BALANCE 31ST DECEMBER 1989		£3,358		£2,353

REPORT OF THE AUDITORS
TO THE MEMBERS OF THE MANCHESTER MEDICAL SOCIETY

We have audited the financial statements on pages 20 to 24 in accordance with approved Auditing standards.

In our opinion the financial statements give a true and fair view of the Society's affairs as at December 31st, 1989 and of the surplus for the year ended on that date.

ROBERTS & CO
Chartered Accountants

4th Floor
John Dalton House
121 Deansgate
Manchester
M3 2AR

April 25th, 1990

Honorary Librarian's Report
For the Session 1989-90

In the John Rylands University Library the major task of reorganising the locations of the periodical holdings has been completed with the Biological Sciences periodicals funded by the Science and Medicine sections of the Library being shelved together. The structural repairs in Area 3 (Medical Periodicals) are also finished.

By the end of the session the review of the periodicals holdings should be finalised. When the exercise began it was intended that there would be some cancellations in order to commence subscriptions to other periodicals more relevant to the needs of current users. Unfortunately a major reduction in Library funding has led to a request for reductions in the periodicals subscriptions far beyond that originally envisaged. The Medical Library Committee is aware of the strong feelings of the members on this matter and has tried to balance the varied interests of the different groups of users. A list of titles for cancellation will be considered by the Medical Library Committee before any action is taken by the Library. Although many titles in the John Rylands University Library are also taken by hospital libraries there is no guarantee that this will continue but it is hoped that the NHS and University libraries will liaise in order to maintain the variety of periodicals which have been available to members of the Society.

It is with regret that I announce the retirement from the Medical Library Committee of Professor A R Hunter and Dr S Oleesky. They have both given long and valuable service to the Committee and I wish to record the committee's appreciation and thanks for their contributions. The committee was also sorry to hear of the resignation of Mrs Patricia Bowden who provided secretarial assistance and wished to express its appreciation of her work.

In conclusion, I wish to thank Mrs Valerie Ferguson, the Medical Librarian of the John Rylands University Library for her help throughout the year.

ANN FELICITE TUXFORD
Honorary Librarian

Section of Medicine

Office-bearers and Members of the Council for the Session 1990-91:

PRESIDENT
Colin Bray

IMMEDIATE PAST PRESIDENT
Frank Ian Lee

PRESIDENT ELECT
John Perkins

HONORARY SECRETARY
William James Kenneth Cumming

COUNCIL
David Coussmaker Anderson
Roy Bridson Clague
Michael John Goodman
Michael Steven Hendy
Venkateswaren Mani
John Paul Miller
David Spurr
William Philip Stephens
Humberto Juan Testa
Thomas Walter Warnes

Report for the Session 1989-90

The Section held four meetings during the year of which two were joint meetings. Unfortunately the prize evening had to be cancelled due to insufficient entries but is hoped that one will be held during the next session. The joint meeting with the North West Region Association of Physicians was held at the Manchester Royal Infirmary and the other meetings were held in the Stopford Building of the University of Manchester. This format will change next session as it is planned to hold some of the meetings outside the city centre. Membership of the Section remains constant at 330. The full programme was as follows:

1989
October 4th
Presidential Address
Dr F I LEE   Vinyl chloride induced liver disease

November 1st
Joint Meeting with the North West Regional Association of Physicians
Professor W I MACDONALD   The dynamics of multiple sclerosis

1990
February 7th
Joint Meeting with the Section of Pathology
Dr A B PRICE   Iatrogenic and autogenic diseases of the gastro-
                                    intestinal tract

March 7th
Research Topics

Dr F W BALLARDIE — Progressive IgA nephropathy - advances in pathogenesis and treatment

Dr J R E DAVIS — In vitro studies of human pituitary tumours

Dr P O'NEILL — Geriatric Medicine

Professor R C TALLIS — Epilepsy in old age

Section of Surgery

Office-bearers and Members of the Council for the Session 1990-91:

PRESIDENT
Robin James Barnard

VICE PRESIDENT
Humfrey John Done

IMMEDIATE PAST PRESIDENT
William George Thompson Bell

HONORARY SECRETARY
Edward Smalley Kiff

COUNCIL
John Bancewicz
Brian David Hancock
Roger James Williams
Martin Cooper Wilson

Report for the Session 1989-90

The Section had an enjoyable and instructive year and both meetings and dinners have been well attended. The ICI Registrar's Prize evening was once more to a very high standard. This session Dr Patterson, International Director for ICI was able to attend. The Prize was awarded to Miss Rosalind Page. The programme finished with a joint meeting with the Royal College of Surgeons of Edinburgh. The chosen topic kept the audience and speakers talking well into the night. The Section looks forward to seeing more new members at next sessions meetings. Membership of the Section has increased again to 278 and the full programme was as follows:

1989
October 10th
Presidential Address
Mr W G T BELL

Identity, role and changing patterns of treatment in Stockport

November 14th
Professor A JOHNSON

Shattering news for gallstones - implications for new treatments

December 12th
Mr J CRAVEN

Gastric cancer

1990
January 9th
Mr R J NICHOLLS

Rectal cancer

February 13th
Michael Boyd Memorial Lecture
Mr P L HARRIS

Reconstructive arterial surgery - expectations past and present

27

March 13th
ICI Surgical Registrars' Prize Evening

Mr G ASKEW — Delay in presentation and misdiagnosis of strangulated hernia: a prospective study

Miss ROSALIND PAGE — Thalamotomy for levodopa induced dyskinesia

Mr M L PANTELIDES — Photodynamic therapy for localised prostatic cancer: laser light penetration in the human prostate gland

Mr I A TRAIL — Adhesives in tendon repair

Mr R VOHRA — Effect of shear stress imposed by flow on endo-thelial cell mono-layers on ePTFE comparing preclot and fibronectin matrices

April 10th
Symposium
Mr B HEGARTY, QC
Mr P REVINGTON — Medical/Legal problems
Dr G J ROBERTS

May 9th
Joint Meeting with Royal College of Surgeons of Edinburgh
Mr A H ROSTHORN — Controversies surrounding Hess's death - who
Mr W H THOMAS — was he?

Section of Pathology

Report for the Session 1989-90

Seven meetings were held during the session including the joint meeting with the Section of Medicine. The Section continues the tradition of holding a dinner in the Refectory of the University after the meetings to which all members are invited to attend and bring guests if they wish. The Trainee Medal for this session was presented to Jane M Edwards. The standard of entries was very high and the judges complimented all the entrants on their papers. The membership of the Section remains fairly constant at 236. The full programme for the session was as follows:

1989
October 11th
Professor P VADGAMA — Biosensors

November 8th
Professor R W LACEY — The microbial hazards of food consumption

December 13th
Dr J H SCARFFE — The clinical role of haemopoietic growth factors

1990
January 10th
T D ALLEN PhD DSc — Time lapse and ultrastructural studies of living bone marrow

February 7th
Joint Meeting with the Section of Medicine
Dr A B PRICE — Latrogenic and autogenic diseases of the gastro-intestinal tract.

March 14th
Papers for the Trainee's Medal in Pathology

Dr ALISON DUFFY — A new low density lipoprotein assay

Dr JANE EDWARDS — Squamous cell carcinoma of the oesophagus - the prognostic significance of various histological criteria, DNA Ploidy and intraepithelial neoplasia

Dr R J HALE — Prognostic factors in uterine cervical carcinoma

Dr K G KERR — Four hour identification of Listeria species

Dr P K MACCALLUM — Reduction of factor VIIIC, a risk factor for ischaemic heart disease, by fixed dose Warfarin

Dr N WILKINSON — C-erb B2 oncogene expression in lung and ovarian tumours

April 11th
Presidential Address

Dr M HARRIS — Diagnosing lymphomas - then and now

Section of Anaesthesia

Office-bearers and Members for the Council for the Session 1990-91:

PRESIDENT
John Michael Anderton

PRESIDENT-ELECT
Finlay Nicol Campbell

IMMEDIATE PAST PRESIDENT
Edward Alan Shaw

HONORARY SECRETARIES
Eileen Lesley Horsman
Janette Johnston Brown

COUNCIL
Anne Elizabeth Dingwall
Christine Mary Earlam
Stephen George Greenhough
Jill Hargreaves
Abdul Hassanet Mohammed Mollah
Glenys Phillips
Bernard Reginald Puddy
Christopher Lewis Tolhurst-Cleaver
David Kenneth Whitaker

Report for the Session 1989-90

A total of seven meetings were held during the session. The joint meeting with the Liverpool Society of Anaesthetists was held in Manchester and the final meeting of the session was held at the Preston Post-graduate Centre. The ICI and Abbott prize evening attracted a large number of entries and they were all of a very high standard. This year the ICI Prize went to Dr Denise G Stott and the Abbott Prize to Dr Gillian M Field. At the end of the session the Section changed its name from the Section of Anaesthetics to the Section of Anaesthesia. Membership of the Section has risen slightly to 209. The full programme was as follows:

1989
October 12th
Presidential Address
Dr E A SHAW   The anaesthetist and paediatric oncology

November 9th
Air Commodore C A B McLAREN   Aspects of aviation medicine or does flying
                                         injure your health?

December 14th
Professor P HUTTON   The evolution of anaesthetic monitoring

1990
January 11th
Dr P MORRIS   Anaesthesia and Duchenne Dystrophy-a model
                                         for clinical audit

February 8th
Papers for the ICI and Abbott Registrars' Prizes

Dr GILLIAN M FIELD	Epidural analgesia in labour - a comparison using the T12/L1 and the L3.4 interspace
Dr K G LEE	Effect of tube resistance on alveolar pressure during simulated one-lung ventilation
Dr DENISE G STOTT	The analgesic and respiratory depressant effects of a variety of opiates in mice
Dr N M TIERNEY	Propofol anaesthesia for cardiac catheterization in children

March 15th
Joint Meeting with the Liverpool Society of Anaesthetists (in Manchester)

Dr M J BEECH	Mass spectrometry: today, tomorrow, never?
Dr T D RYAN	In utero transfer - the forgotten patient

April 5th
Symposium
Dr A HUFTON
Dr K MOORE   Anaesthesia and laser surgery
Dr J SHAW

Section of Odontology

Office-bearers and Members of the Council for the Session 1990-91:

PRESIDENT
Peter Roland White

VICE PRESIDENT AND PRESIDENT ELECT
Geoffrey Owen Taylor

IMMEDIATE PAST PRESIDENT
Ben David Cohen

HONORARY SECRETARY
Alison Jane Elizabeth Qualtrough

HONORARY EDITOR
Philip Sloan

HONORARY TREASURER
David John Eldridge

COUNCIL
Philip Alan Banks
David Cunningham
David John Hillary
Iain Campbell Mackie
James Fraser McCord
Mark Roy Trevelyan

Report for the Session 1989-90

During the session six general meetings were held in the Architecture Building. A buffet dinner was held after five of the meetings but in April, to coincide with the Annual General Meeting of the Section, a dinner was held in the University Refectory. The Alan Hilton Medal was awarded to Mr C Irwin. The prize is awarded annually and papers are invited from members who have not previously read a paper. At the Annual General Meeting two members, Pamela Hobson and John Hamilton Howarth, were made Honorary Members in recognition of their contribution to the Section. Membership remains fairly steady at 147 and the full programme was:

1989
October 30th
Presidential Address
Mr B D COHEN   Piggy in the middle

November 27th
Mr G KENT   Dentist/patient communication - participation
                                       workshop

1990
January 29th
Alan Hilton Medal and Members' Evening
Mr P R GREEN   Exciting new developments in Periodontal
                                       Therapy

Mr C IRWIN

Modulation of gingival connective tissue during the inflammatory response

Mr M MCGURK

A growth factor in human saliva

February 27th
Mr J F MCCORD

Hydroxyapatite and localised ridge augmentation

March 26th
Mr J S ZAMET

The borderland between periodontal disease and the dental pulp

April 30th
Mr J G PHILLIPS

Reconstructive problems in Maxillo-facial surgery

Section of General Practice

Report for the Session 1989-90

The Section has not met during the session but its members were specifically invited to attend two meetings of the Section of Paediatrics.

It is hoped that the Section may be revived during the coming session although the format of meetings may be different.

There are still 162 members of the Section.

Section of Paediatrics

Office-bearers and Members of the Council for the Session 1990-91:

PRESIDENT
John Lancelot Burn

PRESIDENT ELECT
David Ivor Keith Evans

IMMEDIATE PAST PRESIDENT
John Harwood Keen

HONORARY SECRETARY
Sadrudin Kassam Mohamed Jivani

COUNCIL
Steven Walter D'Souza
Angus David Kindley
Shirley Anne Leslie
Richard Ward Newton
Jill Roland
Maurice Super

Report for the Session 1989-90

Four meetings were held during the session including a general symposium. During the session members of the Section were canvassed by questionnaire in an attempt to discover why attendance at meetings is decreasing. The majority of replies came from those who already attend the meetings and they voted, in the main, for few changes to be made apart from a change of venue from time to time. The Council will monitor the situation during the next session and members will be notified of any changes that are proposed.

Discussions were held with the Manchester Paediatric Club, Dr John Couriel, the Post Graduate Tutor and the Department of Child Health in order to improve and co-ordinate the various post graduate meetings being held in Manchester. There is no doubt that the Manchester Paediatric Club and the Section need to collaborate very closely and discussions will be held to this effect. The outcome will be reported to members later. Membership has decreased slightly and stands at 151. The full programme was as follows:

1989
October 19th
Symposium

Mr A BIANCHI	Neonatal repair of cleft lip and palate
Mr A DICKSON	Surgical philosophy in gastro-intestinal reflux
Miss C M DOIG	Inflammatory bowel disease
Mr D GOUGH	Progress with plastic in paediatric urology

36

December 14th
Dr J R SIBERT

New hope in preventing childhood accidents

1990
February 15th
Dr J P R JENKINS

Magnetic resonance imaging in children

April 19th
Presidential Address
Dr J H KEEN

"Dear Dr..." - children as out-patients

Section of Psychiatry

Report for the Session 1989-90

The pattern of holding six meetings during the session was continued and attendance has been good. The topics chosen by the speakers were both interesting and varied. Members of the Section are reminded that the dinner following the lectures are open to them and their guests. Membership of the Section has increased slightly to 131. The full programme was as follows:

1989
October 24th
Dr J A STRANG — The impact of A.I.D.S. on drug misuse: policy and practice

November 21st
Professor A C P SIMS — The phenomenology of neurosis

1990
January 30th
Dr J HIGGINS — A psychiatrist on the Parole Board

February 27th
Professor C A BUTTERWORTH — Psychiatric nursing out of control

March 27th
Professor W I N KESSEL — Abandonment of leadership: the stance of the modern psychiatrist

April 24th
Presidential Address
Dr A A CAMPBELL — Forensic psychiatry in the North West

Section of Public Health Medicine

Office-bearers and Members of the Council for the Session 1990-91:

PRESIDENT
Ian Maxwell Leck

PRESIDENT ELECT
David Hughes Vaughan

IMMEDIATE PAST PRESIDENT
William Peter Povey

HONORARY SECRETARY
Ian Frederick Greatorex

COUNCIL
Robert Bullough
Christopher Paul Hallett
Lorraine Lesley Lighton
Gillian Elizabeth Painter
Morven Roxby
Sabapathy Sivayoham

Report for the Session 1989-90

Six general meetings and a Social event were held during the session. All the general meetings were held in the Medical School of the University of Manchester. 56 members and their guests attended the Social event in July which was a visit to Manchester Town Hall where members were welcomed by the Lord Mayor. The wel visit was followed by a meal at the Kwok Man Restaurant in Chinatown. Although attendance at some meetings was disappointing most of the meetings were reasonably well attended. All the speakers gave thought provoking and interesting addresses on the issues, past and present, relevant to the public health.

The Annual General Meeting of the Section in April changed the name of the Section from Community Medicine to that of Public Health Medicine. Membership of the Section has dropped slightly to 115. The full programme was as follows:

1989
October 26th
Presidential Address
Dr S R PALMER   Food poisoning

November 23rd
Professor C CHANTLER   Resource management and clinical directors

1990
January 25th
Presidential Address
Dr W P POVEY   The Manchester and Salford Lying-in Charity and
                                 the St Mary's Hospitals. A Bi-Centennial Tribute

February 22nd
Professor VALERIE BERAL

The role of epidemiology in the 1980's in Great Britain

March 22nd
Presentations of Work in Community Medicine

Dr P M DARK

Hepatitis B virus infection: which vaccine?

Dr LISA A DAVIES

Meningitis: why bother notifying?

Dr D HUDSON

The impact of A.I.D.S. on intravenous drug users

April 26th
Professor R W LACEY

Food hygiene into the 1990's - public health issues

The offices of the Society are situated in the John Rylands University Library. To reach them, enter the building by the main entrance on Burlington Street. Turn left (past the "New Books" display), left again through the passage to the doorway marked "Staircase and Lift". Take the lift to floor 2M (Area 3). On leaving the lift go straight ahead through the narrow door and passage, and walk the full length of the Law Library to the top of the stairs. The Fellows' Room and the three general offices of the Society are all grouped around the landing area. The office is normally open as follows: Monday - Thursday 9.30am to 5pm, Friday 9.30am to 4.30pm.

The Medical Library is situated in the John Rylands University Library in the same area as the offices of the Society but on the floor below. During term-time and Easter vacation the Library will normally be open: Monday to Friday from 0900 to 2130 hours and Saturday from 0900 to 1300 hours. During Christmas and Summer vacations it will be open: Monday to Friday from 0900 to 1730 hours and Saturday from 0900 to 1300 hours. In addition study and reading facilities are available on Saturdays and Sundays during the Michaelmas and Lent terms from 1300 to 1800 hours. These facilities are also available during the Summer term up to the end of the exam period from 1300 to 2130 hours and on the Spring Bank Holiday from 0900 to 2130 hours.

Books and services may only be obtained on presentation of a current library card. Fellows who do not have a card should apply to the Medical Society offices for a voucher. A reasonable charge is made for certain services including photo-copying and Medline searches.

The Medical Library Committee welcomes suggestions for the purchase of books and periodicals.

Telephone Nos:

MANCHESTER MEDICAL SOCIETY **061-273 6048**
University Internal   3765/66/67

LIBRARY:
Loans Enquiries (Main Counter)   061-275 3717
Information Office   061-275 3751
Medical Librarian   061-275 3729
Inter-Library Loans   061-275 3741
General Information   061-275 3738

UNIVERSITY (All Departments)   061-275 2000
MEDICAL SCHOOL (after 5pm)   061-275 5018
REFECTORY (after 5pm)   061-273 6262

MEDICINE AND INDUSTRIAL SOCIETY

*A history of hospital development in
Manchester and its region 1752–1946*
by
John V Pickstone
University of Manchester

In one of the first histories of its kind, John Pickstone
offers a comprehensive and revealing account of the
two centuries of medical care preceding the National
Health Service. The importance of Manchester as the
classic industrial city, and the variety of urban cultures
in its satellite towns make this region an ideal base for a
study of the economic, social and political factors
affecting hospital development. John Pickstone has
been able to draw on a wealth of original sources and
provides a fascinating reconstruction both of a region's
hospitals and of the national negotiations which
produced the NHS.

This book is of interest not only to historians and those
directly involved in health care; it will offer new insights
to all who wish to improve their understanding of our
society's institutions.

The retail price of this book, which has been published
by the Manchester University Press, is £45.00, but
Fellows of the Society can obtain copies at a special
price of £20.00 (plus £1.00 for postage and packing)
from the Society's offices.

KEY DEADLINE DATES IN THE ANNUAL CYCLE OF THE SOCIETY

	Sections	*Society*
Before the end of JANUARY	Convene meeting of the Council to agree nominations for office-bearers and members of Council for ensuing year.	
FEBRUARY	Convene meeting of Council to arrange programme for forthcoming year.	Convene meeting of the Council to agree nominations for office-bearers of Council for ensuing year.
MARCH	Issue notice giving at least four weeks notice of date of Annual General Meeting of Section.	
APRIL	Annual General Meeting of Section.	Issue notice giving at least four weeks notice of date of Annual General Meeting of Society.
MAY	Negotiate with speakers and prepare Annual Report	Annual General Meeting of Society. Convene meeting of new Council to discuss programme for ensuing year.
JUNE	Finalise details of programme for coming session.	Negotiate with speakers, determine programme of meetings for forthcoming year and prepare Annual Report.
JULY		Check proof of Annual Report and add late details of speakers and titles.
AUGUST		
SEPTEMBER		Circulate printed copies of Annual Report along with October card.
OCTOBER to MAY	Review arrangements for each month: advise MMS office of guests attending dinners. Provide minutes of meetings for typing and filing by office staff.	Circulate copies of monthly programme card and Section dinner invitations etc.

The above timetable, based upon experience over the years, is published here for ready reference by all concerned—particularly by officers and members of the Councils of the Sections of the Society.

RORY F McCLOY
Honorary Secretary

SOME MANCHESTER DOCTORS...

*A biographical collection
to mark the 150th anniversary of*

THE MANCHESTER MEDICAL SOCIETY

edited by
Willis J. Elwood and A. Félicité Tuxford

Manchester University Press has published, on behalf of the Manchester Medical Society, this important and absorbing study commemorating the lives of twenty-four eminent Manchester doctors.

Aimed at the general reader with an interest in medical history, and written by thirty-six contributors (including Sir Douglas Black and Sir Harry Platt), this volume contains commemorative biographies of, among others—Joseph Jordan, Sir James MacKenzie, John Launcelot Burn and Sir John Charnley. They are prefaces with introductory chapters outlining the history and development of the Manchester Medical Society and an appendix containing notes on over 130 other doctors.

Fellows of the Society may obtain a copy from the Society's office at a special price of £5.00 (plus £1.00 p & p).